Psychology and Diabetes Care

Katharine D. Barnard
Cathy E. Lloyd
Editors

Psychology and Diabetes Care

A Practical Guide

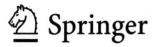 Springer

Editors

Katharine D. Barnard Ph.D.,
CPsychol.
Faculty of Medicine
University of Southampton
Enterprise Road
Southampton Science Park
Chilworth, Southampton, UK

Cathy E. Lloyd Ph.D.
Faculty of Health & Social Care
The Open University
Walton Hall
Milton Keynes, UK

ISBN 978-0-85729-572-9   e-ISBN 978-0-85729-573-6
DOI 10.1007/978-0-85729-573-6
Springer London Dordrecht Heidelberg New York

A catalogue record for this book is available from the British Library

Library of Congress Control Number: 2011945615

Springer is part of Springer Science+Business Media (www.springer.com)

Preface

Welcome to Psychology and Diabetes Care: A Practical Guide!

Diabetes is considered to be a major public health issue in the twenty-first century; however, it is much more than that. Representing a very personal daily challenge for people living with the condition and their families, diabetes requires high levels of self-management to maintain optimal diabetes control and prevent or delay the onset of long-term diabetes-related complications. For some people, this challenge can become demanding and burdensome, leading to feelings of burnout and despair. This challenge continues with no respite or cure available. Yet the experience of living with diabetes can vary dramatically from person to person. People are all unique and adapt to and behave differently in any given situation. The personal response to diabetes is no different. Positive psychological adjustment to the condition is crucial, however, to ensure optimal quality of life as well as biomedical outcomes.

The outlook for diabetes care has never been brighter. Advances in technologies, diagnostic screening and improvements in structured education have been immense over the past few years with no sign of such progress abating. Developments in insulin delivery and continuous glucose-monitoring systems mean that people have greater control over their diabetes today than ever before. The amazing achievements of role models with diabetes in sports, the media, and entertainment, to name but a few, illustrate that diabetes does not have to hold people back. The other side of the coin, however, is that people with diabetes and their families are under ever-increasing pressure to maintain optimal self-care behaviors and take greater responsibility for healthy lifestyle choices than ever before.

Throughout the following chapters, each author explores a different aspect of diabetes and positive adjustment to it. We have tried to provide a balance between psychological theory, research, and practical experience. As such, there are practical tips throughout the chapters designed to help you support people with diabetes more effectively, and it is hoped that you will use the book as a handy resource to pick up and refer to whenever you need to. Providing the information that people need at a time and way that is most appropriate to them is key to optimizing diabetes care and enhancing quality of life. Balancing short-term situations with longer term objectives using the behavior change techniques presented in this book will help provide the support required for living with diabetes.

The book starts by taking a look at the diagnosis of diabetes and considers what that might mean to the individual, as well as some of the common psychological problems associated with diabetes such as depression and burnout. Chapter 2 contains two very open, honest, and personal stories from two people living with diabetes and their journey from diagnosis to the present day. It is important to keep in mind that these are only two individual personal stories and not everybody with diabetes will have similar experiences. This chapter is a very useful one though, because it reminds us of the range of emotions that people can experience as they work through their diagnosis and come to terms with their condition. Chapters 3 and 4 look at how diabetes is experienced in children and adolescents, and gives practical advice on how to support these groups and their families through the specific stages of change as they move into adulthood. Here we take a look at some of the social challenges that can be associated with living with diabetes, with a specific focus on the impact of alcohol on social relationships and diabetes self-management. There are some very useful tips to help health care practitioners talk openly about potentially difficult issues both within and beyond clinic settings.

Chapter 5 focuses on what we have called "special groups," the first of which considers the particular concerns for individuals from minority ethnic groups, using South Asians with diabetes as an example. The second special group discussed is women experiencing pregnancy and looks at the needs of women through pre-conception care and gestational diabetes and, in particular, the psychological impact of increased risk and increased monitoring. The psychological impact of having more than one condition – often termed "comorbidity" – is the focus of the next section, with the chapter finishing with a consideration of the particular psychological needs of older people with diabetes.

Finally, Chapters 6 and 7 look at psychological behavior change techniques to help support people with diabetes in clinical settings, giving some useful practical examples. While supporting optimal diabetes care requires a multidisciplinary team approach, the major contributor to optimal diabetes control is the person living with the condition. Only they know whether they are able or willing to attempt the behavior changes necessary to maximize well-being and good diabetes control and, as such, are an essential part of that team.

We hope this book gives you an in-depth understanding of the experiences of people with diabetes and will be a useful ongoing resource, providing you with some practical tips on giving psychological support to individuals with this serious long-term condition. This book is the result of many different people's hard work and we would like to take this opportunity to thank them all. In particular, a vote of thanks goes to all our colleagues who contributed to this book and to our editorial assistants at Springer, Denise Roland and Teresa Dudley.

Contributor Biographies

Dr. Lorraine Albon graduated in medicine in 1992 after first completing a degree in human sciences. Her internal medicine training was undertaken in London and Birmingham, where she developed an interest in diabetes and endocrinology. Her subspecialty interests include obesity management and adolescent care. She completed her M.Sc. in 1999 with distinction, and in 2004 was appointed as consultant physician in Portsmouth. She has multiple roles; primarily an acute physician, she has developed her diabetes service with a focus on bariatric medicine; she is also the lead for care of young people with diabetes in the Gosport area of Hampshire. A lecturer on issues pertaining to young people at the University of Warwick, Dr. Albon also speaks locally and regionally on both obesity and young people's issues. She is currently involved with both the Society for Acute Medicine and the Royal College of Physicians with the aim of improving the experience of young people in the acute sector.

Dr. Katharine Barnard specializes in the psychosocial impact of diabetes. Having attained an Open University honors degree, followed by an M.Sc. in health psychology and a Ph.D. in quality of life in type 1 diabetes at the University of Southampton, Dr. Barnard has a longstanding research interest in the psychosocial issues associated with diabetes. Through this research, a broad understanding has been gained of the factors that contribute to the quality of life and the impact that diabetes has on both the individuals with the condition and their family members. Dr. Barnard's collaborative research spans a number of multinational clinical trials covering psychosocial aspects of diabetes. The effect of diabetes, both medically and socially in terms of everyday coping, psychosocial impact, and psychological burden, is a multifaceted and complex area and Dr. Barnard's research to date has made significant advances in unraveling some of these complexities. Other research interests include maximizing recruitment to clinical trials and self-monitoring of blood glucose in type 2 diabetes. Dr. Barnard is an associated lecturer at a number of UK universities and maintains strong academic links.

Michelle Bushell qualified as a registered nurse in 2008 following completion of a bachelor of science degree in nursing from the former University of Central England in Birmingham. Since qualifying, she has worked as a staff nurse within the acute medicine directorate on a ward with a specialty in diabetes. Michelle was diagnosed with type 1 diabetes at the age of 10 in November 1994 following a rapid onset of symptoms and has been privy to many advances over the years in treatment regimes. Michelle believes the decision in choosing her career path of becoming a diabetes specialist nurse is due to the outstanding care she has received over the years and would like to be able to contribute that similar care to fellow patients with diabetes. Michelle is passionate about improving diabetes care and is a regular guest speaker on the Warwick University Certificate in Diabetes Care Course and has recently completed her postgraduate diabetes degree course herself at Birmingham City University.

Dr. Deborah Christie is a consultant clinical psychologist and honorary reader in pediatric and adolescent psychology. She is clinical lead for pediatric and adolescent psychology at University College London Hospitals NHS Foundation Trust. She currently works with young people who are searching for ways to live with chronic illness, including diabetes, obesity, arthritis, chronic fatigue, and chronic pain syndromes. She has published over 80 peer-reviewed papers and chapters. Her current research interests include neuropsychological outcomes in children and adolescent survivors of meningitis, quality of life measures in chronic illness, and the development of effective multidisciplinary interventions for diabetes and obesity in children and adolescents. Dr. Christie is an established international presenter and trainer in motivational and solution-focused therapies, helping multidisciplinary teams develop effective communication skills with adolescents and families. She developed the Healthy Eating Lifestyle Programme (HELP) as part of the University College Hospital Weight Management Clinic. In 2001, Dr. Christie was awarded the Association for the Study of Obesity Best Practice Award and the Society for Adolescent Medicine Diabetes Award in Adolescent Health. She received the award for Outstanding Scientific Achievement in Clinical Health Psychology in 2004.

Sue Cradock qualified as a nurse in 1974 at Stoke Mandeville Hospital, UK, and started to develop her career in diabetes after she moved to Portsmouth in 1976. She achieved her diploma in nursing in 1979 and her master's degree in 1997. She then worked with Professor Ken Shaw to develop the Specialist Diabetes Service for Portsmouth from 1985 onward. The team won the Hospital Doctor Diabetes Team of the Year Award in 1998. Sue was appointed as consultant nurse to this service in 2001 until 2010 when she left to pursue her academic career. Sue was also a cofounder of the Royal College of Nursing Diabetes Forum and its chairman from 1990 to 1992. She then joined the Education Committee of the British Diabetic Association (now Diabetes UK) and acted as chairman for a year before the reorganization took place. Sue was a cofounder of the DESMOND program and continues to support the development of structured education through this initiative by being a national trainer and assessor as well as part-time educator. She is part of the team that was awarded the Health Service Journal Skills Development Award in 2007 for the quality assurance work of DESMOND. She has developed specific expertise in the area of "self-management" support and behavior change in those who deliver care to people with diabetes as well as to those who live life with diabetes. She is currently undertaking a funded Ph.D. to study the quality assurance tools used to observe educator behavior in the DESMOND group program. Sue also acts as education consultant to industry and academia.

Joe Fraser was diagnosed with type 1 diabetes in 1999, aged 13. After learning to take control, he wrote *Joe's Rough Guide to Diabetes*, a practical manual for people with type 1 diabetes. In 2006, with sponsorship from Sanofi Aventis, 20,000 copies were published by Wiley and distributed throughout the UK. After completing an English degree at Exeter College, Oxford, in 2008, Joe set up Joe's Diabetes Ltd (www.joes-diabetes.com), rewrote the book for a second edition, and designed "Joe's Small-in-one" carry case. This compact bag takes all a person with type 1 diabetes needs for 24 h treatment, which gives a good reserve of supplies without being too bulky. In 2010, Joe appeared in an article for *The Times* about his diabetic experiences and became involved with various diabetic groups. These include the Warwick Diabetes Research, Education and Users' Group; Getting Sorted; and The SWEET Project and NHS Diabetes, helping to standardize education for patients. This work has led to Joe giving talks on diabetes to diabetic groups, schools, universities, and at the Diabetes UK Conference in 2011.

Dr. Colin Greaves is a senior research fellow at the Peninsula College of Medicine and Dentistry (Primary Care), specializing in research on lifestyle behavior change. He is a chartered psychologist and a practitioner health psychologist. He is engaged in a wide range of research to develop and evaluate practical interventions to help people change their lifestyle behaviors in order to reduce their risk of cardiovascular disease and type 2 diabetes. Dr. Greaves has also helped to develop intervention materials and training courses for service providers to support people to lose weight (through changes in diet and physical activity) and to stop smoking. He helped to develop a European guideline (the IMAGE guideline) on the prevention of type 2 diabetes and its associated training curriculum for diabetes prevention managers.

Professor Richard Holt trained at the University of Cambridge and the London Hospital Medical College. He undertook his postgraduate training in diabetes and endocrinology in the South East Thames Region. While a Medical Research Council Clinical Training Fellow, he completed a Ph.D. on the growth hormone – insulin-like growth factor axis in childhood liver disease. He was appointed as senior lecturer in endocrinology and metabolism at the University of Southampton in May 2000, was promoted to reader in March 2006, and became professor in diabetes and endocrinology in September 2008. Richard's current research interests are broadly focused around clinical diabetes and endocrinology. These encompass studies of the relationship between mental illness and diabetes, the developmental origins of adult diabetes and cardiovascular disease, and the effects of the adult environment, in particular the benefits of physical activity and risk of obesity. Richard is currently the European region editor of *Diabetic Medicine* and reviews editor of *Diabetes, Obesity and Metabolism*. He is the chair of the Council of Healthcare Professionals of Diabetes, UK, having previously served as the vice chair of the Science & Research Group and chair of the Annual Professional Conference Organising Committee.

Dr. Cathy Lloyd is an academic and researcher at the Open University, where she is a senior lecturer in the Faculty of Health & Social Care. She has been involved in teaching pre-registration nursing and courses in health care studies, where understanding the personal experience of diabetes and other long-term conditions is a central tenet. Her current research interests include the experience of comorbid physical and mental illness, and, in particular, the impact of the ever-increasing burden of diabetes and its psychological sequelae on both an individual as well as societal level. Recently, the measurement of psychological well-being and the cultural applicability of existing tools to measure psychological distress in minority ethnic groups has been the focus of her funded research, which has led her to international collaborations with colleagues from the Dialogue on Diabetes and Depression (DDD) as well as from the European Association for the Study of Diabetes (EASD) Psychosocial Aspects Study Group.

Professor Alan Sinclair is an international expert in diabetes and geriatrics and is professor of medicine at the University of Bedfordshire and dean at the Bedfordshire & Hertfordshire Postgraduate Medical School. He regularly provides advice for the UK NICE organization and for the Department of Health on matters relating to diabetes in older people. He has produced international guidelines on diabetes care for older people available at www.instituteofdiabetes.org. Professor Sinclair was academic director of the EUGMS (European Union Geriatric Medicine Society) between 2001 and 2005. He has interests in ageing and nutrition, stroke illness, and cognitive dysfunction/Alzheimer's disease. He is the lead for diabetes in the GerontoNet collaboration, headed by Professor Vellas of Toulouse. Alan has been designated a WHO Expert in Diabetes. He is the author of many papers in the area of geriatrics, nutrition, and diabetes. He is the author of the first textbook on diabetes in old age published by Wiley & Sons, and in 2009 the third edition of this textbook was published. Professor Sinclair is the national clinical lead in England for diabetes and older people and is currently leading a global initiative on diabetes in older people for the EASD. In May 2008, Professor Sinclair officially launched the first institute of its kind devoted to diabetes in older people (Institute of Diabetes for Older People, IDOP) and has assembled a prestigious advisory board to promote its development.

Contents

List of Contributors

Lorraine Albon, M.B.B.S., M.Sc, FRCP Medical
Assessment Unit and Diabetes/Endocrinology Department,
Queen Alexandra Hospital, Portsmouth Hospitals
NHS Trust, Portsmouth, Hampshire, UK

Katharine D. Barnard, Ph.D., CPsychol. Faculty of
Medicine, University of Southampton,
Enterprise Road, Southampton Science Park, Chilworth,
Southampton, UK

Michelle Bushell, B.Sc. (Hons) Nursing RN Department
of Acute Medicine – Diabetes Specialty, Heart of England
NHS Foundation Trust, Birmingham, West Midlands, UK

Deborah Christie, B.Sc., Ph.D., Dip. Clin. Psych. Child
and Adolescent Psychological Services, University College
London Hospitals NHS Foundation Trust, London, UK

Sue Cradock, M.Sc. Department of Health and Sciences,
University of Leicester, Hampshire, England

Joseph J.M. Fraser, B.A. Oxon Joe's Diabetes Ltd,
London, UK

Colin Greaves, Ph.D., CPsychol. Peninsula College
of Medicine and Dentistry, University of Exeter,
Exeter, Devon, UK

Richard I.G. Holt, M.A., M.B., BChir., Ph.D., FRCP, FHEA Human Development and Heath Academic Unit, Faculty of Medicine, University of Southampton, Southampton General Hospital, Southampton, UK

Cathy E. Lloyd, Ph.D. Faculty of Health & Social Care, The Open University, Walton Hall, Milton Keynes, UK

Alan Sinclair, M.Sc., M.D., FRCP Institute of Diabetes for Older People, Beds & Herts Postgraduate Medical School, Bedfordshire, UK

Chapter 1
Psychological Burden of Diabetes and What It Means to People with Diabetes

Katharine D. Barnard, Cathy E. Lloyd, and Richard I.G. Holt

1.1 Introduction

Diabetes mellitus is a complex metabolic disorder character-ized by persistent hyperglycemia (higher than normal blood glucose levels) resulting from defects in insulin secretion, insulin action, or both. It is one of the commonest long-term

K.D. Barnard (✉)
Faculty of Medicine,
University of Southampton, Enterprise Road,
Southampton Science Park, Chilworth,
Southampton, SO16 7NS, UK
e-mail: k.barnard@soton.ac.uk

C.E. Lloyd
Faculty of Health & Social Care,
The Open University, Walton Hall, Milton Keynes, MK7 6AA, UK
e-mail: c.e.lloyd@open.ac.uk

R.I.G. Holt
Human Development and Heath Academic Unit, Faculty of Medicine,
University of Southampton, Southampton General Hospital,
Southampton, UK

K.D. Barnard and C.E. Lloyd (eds.), *Psychology and Diabetes Care*,
DOI 10.1007/978-0-85729-573-6_1,
© Springer-Verlag London Limited 2012

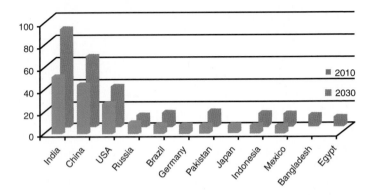

FIGURE 1.1 Prevalence of diabetes in people aged 20–79 in 2010 and projected prevalence in 2030. The ten countries with the highest numbers of people with diabetes are listed (*Source*: IDF Diabetes Atlas 2009)

conditions and represents a major public health burden both in the UK and globally; it is estimated to affect approximately 3.1 million people in the UK alone and approximately 285 million people worldwide [1]. By 2030, it is projected that this figure will rise to more than 435 million as a result of changing population demographics, such as aging and urbanization, changes in lifestyle, such as diet and exercise, and the associated increase in obesity. Figure 1.1 is above provides prevalence figures by country.

Diabetes is not simply a public health burden but rather represents a very personal daily challenge for people living with the condition and their families. This challenge continues with no respite or cure available. Being "diabetic" can have the potential to set people aside from "normal" society and imperceptibly outside the social constructs of what it is to be healthy. These societal norms bring with them prejudices and arbitrary or erroneous rules about how to behave. People with diabetes often report the stigma associated with the condition, affecting not only health but also social functioning [2].

Receiving a diagnosis of diabetes often comes as a shock to the individual and their family, irrespective of whether that diagnosis is of type 1 or type 2 diabetes. This has been likened to the grieving process, whereby individuals and their families may first experience shock, sometimes followed by anger and possibly denial, before the final stage of acceptance [3]. Coping strategies at each stage of this process have consequences for how well people are able to accept the diagnosis and their ability to perform appropriate self-management to maximize good health. The relationship between the person with diabetes and their healthcare team is a vital one, as much new information must be imparted and assimilated, fears about future good health discussed, and new tasks for diabetes self-management learned.

Such new tasks include acceptance of lifestyle change, a new therapy regimen, and self-monitoring of blood glucose by pricking a finger and placing a droplet of blood onto a small strip in a blood glucose meter. For individuals with type 1 diabetes, they must learn how to administer insulin injections to preserve life and, for many, to adjust doses to match carbohydrate intake, while taking into account levels of exercise, illness, or stress.

It is crucial that healthcare professionals have both empathy for and an understanding of the psychosocial needs of people with diabetes alongside the biomedical needs. While technologies and treatments advance, so too a greater awareness of and support for the psychological impact of diabetes is necessary to ensure people are offered appropriate support to complement their self-management. Alongside their new disease status, individuals must also grapple with their new "label" as a "diabetic" and the social, legal, and medical implications that are associated with it. For individuals with type 1 diabetes, they may have the option to register as disabled and must weigh up the benefits and negatives associated with this status.

Appropriate adjustment to diabetes and being able to put the disease into context with other life priorities is essential to avoid being overwhelmed by the condition and feeling controlled by it. Increased treatment flexibility and greater access to education about self-management have enabled people to fit diabetes into their lives rather than vice versa and maintain a balance between respecting the severity of the condition while enjoying both independence and a good quality of life. Living with the daily burden, however, inevitably takes its toll emotionally and psychologically. The way that healthcare professionals provide support and expertise at these times can help ensure positive outcomes both medically and psychosocially. With careful self-management and appropriate medical support, people can minimize the impact of any restrictions and limitations caused by diabetes.

1.2   Cost of Diabetes

The cost of diabetes is both personal and financial. Psychologically, diabetes is demanding, with people with the condition having to perform daily self-management tasks to maintain good health with currently no hope of a cure.

The majority of people with diabetes have type 2 diabetes (approximately 85–90%), with approximately 10–15% of those diagnosed having type 1 diabetes. Type 2 diabetes results from both impaired insulin secretion and resistance to the action of insulin. It is generally diagnosed later in life; however, more recently, people are being diagnosed at earlier ages with this form of diabetes even affecting some adolescents. Type 1 diabetes is caused predominantly by the autoimmune destruction of the insulin-producing β-cells of the pancreatic islets. Worldwide, there are approximately 20 million people with type 1 diabetes. Globally, the incidence and prevalence of type 1 diabetes increased markedly during the second half of the twentieth century. Overall, the incidence rate increased between 3.2% and 5.3% per year during the 1990s, with the most pronounced increase being seen in pre-school children. Most commonly diagnosed in children and adolescents, the average age of onset is around 11 years for girls and 14 years for boys. Increasingly, younger children are being diagnosed with type 1 diabetes with the fastest growing prevalence in the 0–4 year olds. It is anticipated that the prevalence of type 1 diabetes in this age group will increase by 80% by 2020 [4].

This chapter will explore the psychological burden associated with diabetes, from diagnosis through everyday living with the condition to comorbidities of depression, diabetes-related distress, and burnout. It will also give some practical tips for caring for diabetes and its psychological consequences.

1.3   Diagnosis of Diabetes

A diagnosis of diabetes is made if the fasting plasma glucose is ≥7.0 mmol/L (126 mg/dL) or if the random or 2-h glucose tolerance test plasma glucose is ≥11.1 mmol/L (200 mg/dL). The World Health Organization (WHO) and American Diabetes Association have recently expanded the diagnostic criteria to include a glycated hemoglobin (HbA1c) of >6.5% (48 mmol/L) [5]. While a single value is sufficient in an individual with typical symptoms and signs of diabetes, two abnormal values on two separate days are needed in an asymptomatic individual.

The World Health Organization (WHO) diagnostic criteria also recognize two further categories of intermediate abnormal glucose concentrations: impaired fasting glycemia (IFG) and impaired glucose tolerance (IGT), the latter of which can only be diagnosed following a 75-g oral glucose test [6].

1.3.1   Diagnosis of Type 1 Diabetes

Type 1 diabetes is caused by an absolute deficiency of insulin. In populations of white Northern European ancestry, it usually occurs as the result of a T cell–mediated autoimmune destruction of the β-cells of the pancreas. Its presentation and acute complications may be dramatic and may require rapid hospitalization and treatment. Symptoms at diagnosis include extreme thirst, rapid weight loss, and polyuria (the need to urinate frequently). There is currently no cure.

Experience of Type 1 Diagnosis

Tom had been born 7 weeks prematurely and was immediately transferred to the special care baby unit where he recovered well, and the family was looking forward to a long healthy happy life ahead. When Tom was 4 years old, he became unwell over a few weeks, losing a lot of weight and feeling ghastly. Tom's parents took him to their GP and explained the symptoms. Even before the blood test results came back, the sense of doom was palpable, and the results only confirmed the worst news. Tom was referred to the hospital the same day, and the hours passed in a blur of doctors, diagnosis, and dread that he may not survive the next few hours. There were new skills to learn such as how to perform insulin injections, test his blood glucose levels, and learn how to manage diabetes. An endless stream of healthcare professionals came to see Tom and his parents, and a tidal wave of information was forthcoming with folders of more information to take away and read. The doctors kept saying how sorry they were, and Tom's mom wanted to scream at them "that he wasn't dead, although part of her felt like it had died." Eventually, the days passed and they were discharged, with yet more home visits by dieticians and nurses. As the days passed and Tom and his parents became increasingly familiar with the new routines, a tiny light began to emerge slowly at the end of the tunnel, and family life with type 1 diabetes seemed achievable.

1.3.2 Diagnosis of Type 2 Diabetes

Type 2 diabetes has a gradual and insidious onset. The diagnosis is often delayed, and some degree of hyperglycemia may have been present for more than 20 years before the diagnosis is confirmed. Only around 50% of people with type

2 diabetes are diagnosed as a result of the typical diabetes symptoms such as thirst, tiredness, polyuria, and blurred vision. These tend to "creep up" over time and are less dramatic than symptoms experienced by people with type 1 diabetes. The other half is diagnosed as the result of a routine blood test or with the development of a diabetes complication such as eye problems or high blood pressure.

Like type 1 diabetes, type 2 diabetes is associated with premature mortality, predominantly through cardiovascular disease. Even after adjustment for other cardiovascular risk factors, diabetes is associated with a two- to threefold increase in the risk of myocardial infarction or stroke [7].

Experience of Type 2 Diagnosis

Paul was 56 and overweight. For a long time, he had been feeling really tired and lethargic. He had recently remarried, and very soon he and his new wife found out they were expecting a baby. When he accompanied his wife to the antenatal clinic, he realized that some of the questions they were asking applied to him too, and so he went back to his GP to ask for a test for diabetes. His doctor arranged for him to have a glucose tolerance test at the local hospital, which showed that he actually had type 2 diabetes. On hearing this news, Paul was not particularly surprised; after all, both his parents had had diabetes later in life, and he was quite overweight, and he had heard this put you at increased risk for diabetes. Paul was invited back to his GP's to discuss his diagnosis with the practice nurse. He was handed a number of leaflets, including some that looked really worrying which warned him about his risk of blindness, amputations, and heart problems. He decided to wait until he got back home to read these and discuss them with his wife; he knew they would have to start eating more healthily, and perhaps he could take some exercise – he could always push the baby buggy round the park more often.

1.4   Burden of Diabetes

Diabetes is a demanding, long-term condition that impacts not only on the life of the individual but also on the lives of other family members. It can interfere with daily functioning and can cause problems with work, social life, and family relationships. An individual's quality of life is affected not only by the condition but also by the therapy required to manage it [8] which can involve both lifestyle changes and self-management tasks such as self-monitoring of blood glucose. Similarly, the quality of life of family members is affected, with family members reporting limitations and anxiety associated with living with someone with diabetes [9].

1.5   Living with Diabetes

1.5.1   Daily Self-Management and Psychological Burden

There are different daily demands on people with type 1 or type 2 diabetes; however, similarities exist in terms of the chronic nature and incurable aspect of both. For all people with diabetes, there is a relentless daily self-management regimen that requires perseverance in order to maintain optimal health and reduce the risk of long-term complications. For people with type 1 diabetes, there are the demands of frequent self-monitoring of blood glucose, insulin administration, and carbohydrate counting. For people with type 2 diabetes, there are oral medications or insulin injections to take and lifestyle changes such as maintaining weight loss and increasing physical activity.

The knowledge that poor diabetes control can lead to increased risk of diabetes-related complications can, in itself, lead to feelings of stress or diabetes burnout. The added burden of knowing that your ability to self-manage may be directly related to your risk of developing these complications often only exacerbates the enormity of the task.

There can sometimes be a tension between healthcare professionals, whose focus is on medical outcomes and minimizing the risks, and the person with diabetes who may be more concerned with how they manage their daily life and diabetes at the same time. Challenges, such as being able to offer an acceptable meal to the whole family or finding time to exercise in an already busy day, may become important concerns. Healthcare professionals need to understand those tensions and work together with people with diabetes to help solve these issues.

Tips for Supporting Individuals Who Worry About or Are Experiencing the Onset of Long-Term Complications
1. Help patients develop realistic attitudes toward diabetes control.
2. Support patients in realistic expectations for self-management.
3. Help patients work through feelings of guilt that, despite their best efforts, they have been unable to reduce the risks.
4. Provide education and support over the long term to address negative habits and promote positive and confident self-management.

1.5.2 Impact on Social Relationships

As recognized in the (UK) National Service Framework for Diabetes [10], diabetes impacts not only on the individual but also on the health and quality of life of other family members; for example, depression in people with diabetes was associated with increased physical health problems in their families [11]. Similarly, diabetes in at least one of the children may adversely affect the quality of life of other family members [9]. In this latter study, parents' self-reported quality of life was directly affected by the impact of their child's diabetes and treatment regimen. As children grow into young adults, there are further challenges to family life. Young adulthood is a time of increasing responsibility and independence. It is a time of new experiences when young people move away from their parents to university, start a first job, or establish long-term new relationships.

Maintaining "normal" social relationships can also be difficult as the restrictions of achieving good diabetes control are sometimes in direct opposition to societal norms of enjoyment. Take alcohol as an example; although the dangers of alcohol are hotly debated from both a personal and public health perspective, it has played an integral role in almost all human cultures since Neolithic times. All societies, without exception, make use of intoxicating substances, of which alcohol is by far the most common [12]. Drinking places tend to be socially integrative, egalitarian environments, the primary function of which is the facilitation of social bonding. Estimates of alcohol use, alcohol misuse (i.e., associated with harm), and alcohol dependence vary widely; self-reported alcohol use in the general population ranges from 39% to 50% of individuals.

The UK's drinking culture particularly affects young adults and represents a major public health burden and expense to the NHS. Preliminary data indicate alcohol use in young adults with T1DM represent a serious public health problem, although the estimates of the prevalence of misuse vary widely [13, 14]. As medical advice to young people with type 1 diabetes is to drink in moderation, any estimate of alcohol and drug taking is likely to be affected by underreporting by participants who may fear reprisal [15]. Increased access to alcohol, with fewer familial restrictions or monitoring, is associated with increased alcohol consumption and alcohol-associated risk behaviors [14]. The provision of better healthcare to young people with T1DM relies on acceptance that alcohol use occurs and clinicians need to be educated in the management of this underappreciated health issue.

Tips for Managing Social Relationships
1. Recognize the impact of diabetes on family members and others.
2. Understand the role of family in the patient's diabetes care.
3. Offer options so that patients and their families can choose the best care pathway that will suit their lifestyle.

1.6   Diabetes and Depression

Depression is a major, disabling illness affecting 121 million people worldwide. At any one time, one in ten people will suffer mental illness with 450 million people having mental illness globally. By 2030, depression will be the second largest contributor to the global burden of disease. The World Health Organization defines depression as "a common mental disorder that presents with depressed mood, loss of interest or pleasure, feelings of guilt or low self-worth, disturbed sleep or appetite, low energy, and poor concentration." It affects people of all genders, ages, and backgrounds. Ranging from subclinical depressive symptomatology (Table 1.1), at its worst depression can lead to suicide, contributing to an estimated 850,000 deaths worldwide every year [16]. Frequently occurring alongside other physical long-term conditions (e.g., heart disease or diabetes), depression can be reliably diagnosed and treated in primary care, yet fewer than 25% of those affected have access to effective treatment [16].

Primary care–based treatments, such as psychotherapy or antidepressants, although not universally available, are associated with improved quality of care, improved satisfaction with care, improved health functioning and outcomes, and indirectly with improved economic productivity and household wealth. For moderate to severe depression, antidepressants are effective; however, for mild to moderate depression, their effectiveness is less proven. Such treatments, however, are firmly rooted in the medical model of care and rely

TABLE 1.1 Symptoms of depression that may be measured in common self-report instruments used in both research and care

Feeling sad/depressed mood

Inability to sleep

Early waking

Lack of interest/enjoyment

Tiredness/lack of energy

Loss of appetite

Feelings of guilt/worthlessness

Recurrent thoughts about death/suicide

heavily on the prescription of antidepressant medication, the effectiveness of which remains under debate [17, 18].

The prevalence of comorbid depression is significantly higher in individuals with diabetes than the general population, with current epidemiological evidence suggesting that at least one third of people with diabetes also have a lifetime risk of developing clinically relevant depressive disorders [19–21]. People with diabetes are two to three times more likely to be considered to be depressed than people without diabetes [22, 23]. Yet, the relationship appears bidirectional with depression also increasing the risk for diabetes [24], making the scenario "chicken and egg." For example, one research study in the UK reported nearly a fourfold increased risk of diabetes in depressed men and a one-and-a-half-times greater risk of diabetes in depressed women [25]. Furthermore, this latter study found that higher depression scores were associated with both diagnosed and undiagnosed diabetes, suggesting that the link between diabetes and depression does not solely result from the psychological distress experienced with the disease diagnosis. Other antecedents include poor social situation and low birth weight, and thus the relationship between diabetes and depression is complex and has yet to be fully understood.

It has been argued that the unremitting practical and emotional burdens that often accompany diabetes self-management may play an important role in the increased risk for depression [26]. An alternative argument is that depression can lead to poor health behaviors; in people with diabetes this could mean that their daily diabetes self-management might be affected, which may impact on blood glucose levels, potentially increasing the risk of developing diabetes-related complications [27–29] and compromise quality of life [30]. Lower (subclinical) levels of depressive symptoms are also common in people with diabetes, with an estimated prevalence ranging from 31% to 45% in people with diabetes [31, 32]. Whatever their cause or effect, symptoms of depression need to be identified and, where appropriate, treated.

A key issue lies in the assessment of depression as compared to diabetes burnout or diabetes-related distress and the ability to disentangle these symptoms from those of depression. This has serious implications for care and any associated treatment or support. Further research still needs to be carried out to address the personal burden of balancing diabetes (both medical and self-management components) with other competing demands on people's time, energy, and workload in order to reduce this risk [22, 26].

1.7   Depression or Diabetes Burnout?

Subclinical depression is a term used when individuals present with depressive symptoms but do not meet the criteria for a diagnosis of clinical depression. In some recent research conducted in the Netherlands [33], approximately one third of people with type 1 diabetes and 37–43% of people with type 2 diabetes reported symptoms of depression but were not diagnosed with clinical depression. These rates were far higher than the proportion of people who had been given an actual diagnosis of depression. However, individuals with subclinical depression will very often not receive treatment but will (be forced to) cope with their symptoms alone. The impact of this in terms of effect on family, work, social life, and overall quality of life remains unknown to a large extent and is an area where further research is needed.

On the other hand, research has demonstrated that there are a substantial proportion of individuals who are not depressed and do not report depressive symptomatology, yet still feel unable to cope with their diabetes. It has been suggested that these people are experiencing diabetes-related distress or are "burned out" by their diabetes. Diabetes burnout occurs when a person feels "overwhelmed by diabetes and by the frustrating burden of diabetes self-care" [34]. These emotions may be very different to feelings of depression; however, they can still be very destructive and can have serious implications for care.

Symptoms of burnout include:
- Feeling overwhelmed and defeated by diabetes
- Feeling angry about diabetes, frustrated by the self-care regimen, and/or having other strong negative feelings about diabetes
- Feeling that diabetes is controlling their life
- Worrying about not taking care of diabetes well enough yet unable, unmotivated, or unwilling to change
- Avoiding any/all diabetes-related tasks that might give feedback about consequences of poor control
- Feeling alone and isolated with diabetes

Thus, while feelings of diabetes burnout center around feelings about diabetes, depression is a physical and psychological disorder requiring specific medical attention. Treatment options are therefore different for both conditions.

1.8   Financial Costs of Depression and Diabetes

Diabetes represents a major cost in terms of healthcare resources. It is estimated that 10% of the NHS budget is spent on diabetes [35]. This equates to around £9 billion a year (based on 2007/2008 budget for the NHS of approximately £90.7 billion) [36] or

- £173 million a week
- £25 million a day
- £1 million an hour

Breaking these costs down a little, depression is costly in terms of prescriptions per head for all antidepressants increasing 2.8-fold between 1991 and 2002, while the total cost (adjusted for inflation) increased by £310 million. The prescribing of antidepressant drugs has increased relentlessly in recent years, while at the same time there have been growing concerns about the medicalization of human distress and the safety of antidepressant medication [37]. Prescribed medication for depression has been the mainstay of treatment for depression in general practice despite the increasing availability of alternative nonpharmacological psychological therapies such as cognitive behavioral therapy. Increases in the pharmacological treatment of depression have not been matched by the development of psychological services of proved effectiveness [38], and it could be conversely argued that the lack of widespread psychological therapies has driven the large number of prescriptions.

Depression is the strongest predictor of increased hospitalization [39] in individuals with type 1 diabetes, with direct cost implications [40]. Prescribing costs for diabetes and comorbid depression are very high. Figures from the United States indicate that people with diabetes and depression have higher ambulatory care use and greater prescribing than their counterparts without depression [40]. Finally, among individuals with diabetes, total healthcare expenditure for individuals with depression has been shown to be 4.5 times higher than that for individuals without depression [41].

1.9   Screening and Treatments for Depression: A Stepped Care Approach

Validated and reliable measures for depression screening include the Center for Epidemiology Studies Depression (CES-D) scale, the Beck Depression Inventory (BDI), and the Patient Health Questionnaire (PHQ-9). All three of these instruments have been recommended by the National Institute of Health and Clinical Excellence (NICE) as appropriate for use in primary care in the UK [42]. The Hospital Anxiety and Depression scale (HADS) [43] is commonly used to determine the levels of anxiety and depression patients are experiencing. As most people with diabetes are cared for by their primary care physician, it is in this setting that there are key opportunities for screening and providing care for people with mental health issues in their lives.

The current risk of a patient with diabetes suffering from depression can be assessed by the presence or absence of well-known risk factors for depression in diabetes. Depression is more common in patients with diabetes who are female, live alone, experience late or acute complications, and who experienced a critical life event in the past, or had poor glycemic control [44, 45]. Besides the appraisal of risk factors, two verbal screening questions have proved to be effective in detecting unrecognized depression in primary care settings: "During the past month, have you often been bothered by feeling down, depressed, or hopeless?" and "During the past month, have you often been bothered by little interest or pleasure in doing things?" While these two screening questions may be easily administered and quite easily answered by many people attending their GP, this may not be the case for all. It is important to remember that for those whom English is not the first or main language, misunderstanding and confusion may arise. Appropriate services should be put in place therefore to ensure equity of care for all.

The National Institute for Health and Clinical Excellence [46] guidelines for depression services specify clinically proven, best-practice pathways to care via a series of steps, which recognize patient choice and preference (see Fig. 1.2 below). These steps start with watchful waiting and increase in intensity through primary care–led guided self-help and other brief therapies, leading to psychological interventions or medication and eventually to case management and

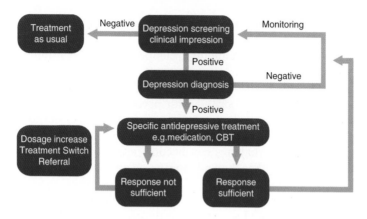

FIGURE 1.2 Stepped care approach in the management of depression in diabetes (Reprinted, with permission of the publisher, from Hermanns and Kulzer, Touch Briefings Ltd. [47])

longer-term specialist treatment. The main aim of a stepped care approach to depression is to simplify the patient pathways, ensure access to more patients, and improve patient well-being. Cost reductions associated with care can be achieved by directing patient referrals, where appropriate, to low-cost community-based treatments first, before progressing to high-cost institutional or specialist services for those who require more intensive support. The notion of improving access to psychological therapies is a concept that is being adopted and adapted across the four UK nations. This is particularly pertinent for the treatment of comorbid depression in diabetes, where the impact of depression has direct and negative consequences for diabetes-related outcomes.

In routine diabetes care, the timely identification of patients with depression seems to be a great challenge; therefore, regular screening for depression is advised by several guidelines [48–50]. Screening tools for depression in diabetes should be simple, have sufficient screening performance, and be acceptable to both healthcare professionals and patients [46].

1.10   Conclusion

Diabetes can be demanding, relentless, and all-consuming. Millions of people live with the condition, and for many it is a manageable, controllable condition. For some people, however, diabetes is associated with psychological burden and can result in diabetes-related distress, depression, or burnout. With appropriate support from healthcare professionals, family, and friends, diabetes can become a manageable part of everyday life rather than all-consuming and controlling life.

Practice implications
- Recognizing and screening for depression is an important aspect of routine care for people with diabetes.
- Diagnosis and treatment of psychological problems can alleviate some of the burden of diabetes.

Key Points
- Diabetes represents a major public health burden both in the UK and globally.
- Comorbid depression is two to three times more prevalent in people with diabetes than the general population.
- Comorbid depression is frequently not considered and is underdiagnosed, in spite of the clinical recommendations.
- Screening, diagnosis, and subsequent treatment of psychological problems are all important for optimal diabetes control and quality of life.

References

1. International Diabetes Federation Diabetes Atlas 2009: website: http://www.idf.org/diabetesatlas/ (2009). Accessed 1 Sept 2011.
2. Barnard K, Lloyd CE. Experiencing depression and diabetes. In: Lloyd CE, Heller TD, editors. Long term conditions; challenges in health and social care. London: Sage Publications; 2011. ISBN 978-0-85702-749-8, 978-0-85702-750-4 (pbk).

3. Bowes S, Lowes L, Warner J, Gregory JW. Chronic sorrow in parents of children with type 1 diabetes. J Adv Nurs. 2009;65((5)):992–1000. doi:10.1111/j.1365-2648.2009.04963.x.

4. Patterson CC, Dahlquist GG, Gyurus E, Green A, Soltesz G. Incidence trends for childhood type 1 diabetes in Europe during 1989–2003 and predicted new cases 2005–20: a multicentre prospective registration study. Lancet. 2009;373:2027–33.

5. American Diabetes Association. Diagnosis and classifications of diabetes. Diabetes Care. 2010;33(1):S62–9.

6. World Health Organisation: Definition, diagnosis and classification of diabetes mellitus and its complications: report of a WHO Consultation, Geneva. WHO/NCD/NCS/99.2; 1999.

7. Graham DJ, Ouellet-Hellstrom R, MaCurdy TE, Ali F, Sholley C, Worrall C, Kelman JA. Risk of acute myocardial infarction, stroke, heart failure, and death in elderly medicare patients treated with rosiglitazone or pioglitazone. JAMA. 2010;304(4):411–8.

8. Rubin R. Diabetes and quality of life. Diabetes Spectr. 2000;3:21.

9. Barnard KD, Speight J, Skinner TC. Quality of life and impact of continuous subcutaneous insulin infusion for children and their parents. Practical Diabetes International. 2008;25:278–283.

10. Department of Health, National service framework for diabetes: standards, crown copyright 2001. http://www.dh.gov.uk/en/Publications and statistics/Publications/PublicationsPolicyAndGuidance/DH_4002951 (2001).

11. Sobieraj M, Williams J, Ryan P. The impact of depression on the physical health of family members. Br J Gen Pract. 1998;48(435):1653–5.

12. The Social Issues Research Centre 'Social and cultural aspects of drinking: a report to the Amsterdam Group'. University of Edinburgh, Edinburgh. www.sirc.org.

13. Glasgow AM, Tynan D, Schwartz R, Hicks JM, Turek J, Driscol C, O'Donnell RM, Getson PR. Alcohol and drug use in teenagers with diabetes mellitus. J Adolesc Health. 1991;12(1):11–4.

14. Ramchandani N, Cantey-Kiser JM, Alter CA, Brink SJ, Yeager SD, Tamborlane WV, Chipkin SR. Self-reported factors that affect glycemic control in college students with type 1 diabetes. Diabetes Educ. 2000;26:656–66.

15. Lee P, Greenfield JR, Campbell LV. Managing young people with Type 1 diabetes in a 'rave' new world: metabolic complications of substance abuse in Type 1 diabetes. Diabet Med. 2009;26(4):328–33.

16. World Health Organisation: Mental health: depression 2010. Website: http://www.who.int/mental_health/management/depression/definition/en/ (2010).

17. Ionnidis J. Effectiveness of antidepressants: an evidence myth constructed from a thousand randomised trials? Philos Ethics Humanit Med. 2008;3:14.

18. Fournier J, et al. Antidepressant drug effects and depression severity. JAMA. 2010;303:47–53.

19. Anderson RJ, Freedland KE, Klaus RE, Lustman PJ. The prevalence of comorbid depression in adults with diabetes: a meta-analysis. Diabetes Care. 2001;24(6):1069–78.

20. Barnard KD, Skinner TC, Peveler R. The prevalence of comorbid depression in adults with Type 1 diabetes. Diabet Med. 2006;23(4): 445–8.

21. Gendelman N, Snell-Bergeon JK, McFann K, Kinney G, Wadwa RP, Bishop F, Rewers M, Maahs DM. Prevalence and correlates of depression in individuals with and without type 1 diabetes. Diabetes Care. 2009;32(4):575–9.

22. Lloyd CE, Hermanns N, Nouwen A, Pouwer F, Underwood L, Winkley K. The epidemiology of depression and diabetes. In: Katon W, Maj M, Sartorius N, editors. Depression and diabetes. Oxford: Wiley-Blackwell; 2010.

23. Pouwer F, Geelhoed-Duijveestihn HLM, Tack CJ, Bazelmans E, Beekman A-J, Heine RJ, Snoek FJ. Prevalence of comorbid depression is high in out-patients with Type 1 or Type 2 diabetes mellitus. Results from the three out-patient clinics in the Netherlands. Diabet Med. 2010;27:217–24.

24. Nouwen A, Winkley K, Twisk J, Lloyd CE, Peyrot M, Ismail K, Pouwer F, for the European Depression in Diabetes (EDID) Research Consortium. Type 2 diabetes mellitus as a risk factor for the onset of depression: a systematic review and meta-analysis. Diabetologia. 2010;53(12):2480–6.

25. Holt RIG, Phillips W, Jameson KA, Cooper C, Dennison EM, Peveler RC. The Hertfordshire Cohort Study Group. Education and psychological aspects: the relationship between depression and diabetes mellitus: findings from the Hertfordshire Cohort Study. Diabet Med. 2009;26:641–8.

26. Pouwer F, Beekman TF, Nijpels G, Dekker JM, Snoek PJ, Kostense RJ, Heine DJ, Deeg DJH. Rates and risks for comorbid depression in patients with Type 2 diabetes mellitus: results from a community-based study. Diabetologia. 2003;46:892–8.

27. Lustman PJ, Anderson RJ, Freedland KE, de Groot M, Carney RM, Clouse RE. Depression and poor glycemic control: a meta-analytic review of the literature. Diabetes Care. 2000;23(7):934–42.

28. Kovacs M, Obrosky DS. Major depressive disorder in youths with IDDM. A controlled prospective study of course and outcome. Diabetes Care. 1997;20(1):45–51.

29. Katon WJ, Rutter C, Simon G, Lin E, Ludman E, Ciechanowski P, Kinder L, Young B, von Korff M. The association of comorbid depression with mortality in patients with type 2 diabetes. Diabetes Care. 2005;28(11):2668–72.

30. Schram MT, Baan CA, Pouwer F. Depression and quality of life in patients with diabetes: a systematic review from the European

depression in diabetes (EDID) research consortium. Curr Diabetes Rev. 2009;5(2):112–9.

31. Gary TL, Crum RM, Cooper-Patrick L, Ford D, Brancati FL. Depressive symptoms and metabolic control in African-Americans with type 2 diabetes. Diabetes Care. 2000;23(1):23–9.

32. Hermanns N, Kulzer B, Krichbaum M, et al. Diabet Med. 2005;22(3):293–300.

33. Pouwer F, Hermanns N. Insulin therapy and quality of life. A review. Diabetes Metab Res Rev. 2009;25 Suppl 1:S4–10.

34. Polonsky W, Anderson B, Lohrer P, Welch G, Jacobson A, Aponte J. Assessment of diabetes related distress. Diabetes Care. 1995;18:754–60.

35. Department of Health: Turning the corner improving diabetes care. 2006. www.dh.gov.uk/en/Publicationsandstatistics/Publications/ PublicationsPolicyAndGuidance/DH_4136141 (2006).

36. NHS Confederation. Key statistics on the NHS. London: NHS Confederation; 2007.

37. Gunnell D, Ashby D. Antidepressants and suicide: what is the balance of benefit and risk? Br Med J. 2004;329:34–8.

38. Hollinghurst S, Kesseler D, Peters TJ, Gunnell D. Opportunity cost of antidepressant prescribing in England: analysis of routine data. Br Med J. 2005;330:999. doi:10.1136/bmj.38377.715799.F7 accessed 15.10.2010.

39. Rosenthal GE, Shah A, et al. Variations in standardized hospital mortality rates for six common medical diagnoses: implications for profiling hospital quality. Med Care. 1998;36(7):955–64.

40. Ciechanowski PS, Katon WJ, Russo JE. Depression and diabetes: impact of depressive symptoms on adherence, function, and costs. Arch Intern Med. 2000;160(21):3278–85.

41. NDST: National diabetes support team fact sheet: no 10: working together to reduce length of stay for people with diabetes. http:// www.diabetologists-abcd.org.uk/Shared_Documents/notice_board/ Factsheet_Payment_By_Results.pdf (2005).

42. NICE: Depression in adults with a chronic physical health problem. http://www.nice.org.uk/nicemedia/live/12327/45865/45865.pdf (2009). Accessed 15 Oct 2010.

43. Zigmond AS, Snaith RP. The hospital anxiety and depression scale. Acta Psychiatr Scand. 2007;67(6):361–70. doi:10.1111/ j.1600-0447.1983.tb09716.

44. Peyrot M, Rubin RR. Diabetes Care. 1997;20(4):585–90.

45. Hermanns N, Kulzer B, Krichbaum M, Kubiak T, Haak T. How to screen for depression and emotional problems in patients with diabetes: comparison of screening characteristics of depression questionnaires, measurement of diabetes-specific emotional problems and standard clinical assessment. Diabetologia. 2006;49(3):469–77.

46. National Screening Committee: The UK's National Screening Committee's criteria for appraising the viability, effectiveness and

appropriateness of a screening programme. Available at: www.nsc. nhs.uk/pdfs/criteria.pdf (2007).

47. Hermanns N, Kulzer B. Diabetes and depression – a burdensome co-morbidity. Eur Endocrinol. 2008;4(2):19–22.

48. ADA. Standards of medical care in diabetes – 2007. Diabetes Care. 2007;30 Suppl 1:S4–41.

49. IDF Clinical Guidelines Task Force. Global guidelines for type 2 diabetes. Brussels: International Diabetes Federation; 2005.

50. Canadian Diabetes Association Clinical Practice Guidelines Expert Committee. Canadian Diabetes Association 2003 clinical practice guidelines for the prevention and management of diabetes in Canada. Can J Diab. 2003;27 Suppl 2:1–152.

Chapter 2
A Patient's Perspective

Michelle Bushell and Joseph J.M. Fraser

Here follows two very different and very personal experiences as told by the individuals themselves about the moment from their diagnosis onwards. The stories contain very personal memories and experiences, and we are very grateful to Michelle and Joe for sharing them. These stories illustrate the personal nature of being diagnosed, and living with diabetes every day. They represent the differences and complexities of human nature and highlight the importance of being aware that for every person with diabetes, how we support their self-management will be different according to their lifestyle and viewpoint.

2.1 Michelle Bushell

Following my diagnosis in November 1994, the changes in diabetes care that I have been privy to have been fairly dramatic. At 10 years old, there is little that can be recalled

M. Bushell (✉)
Department of Acute Medicine – Diabetes Specialty,
Heart of England NHS Foundation Trust,
Bordesley Green East, Bordesley Green,
Birmingham, West Midlands B9 5SS, UK
e-mail: michelle.bushell@heartofengland.nhs.uk

J.J.M. Fraser (✉)
Joe's Diabetes Ltd, Queen's Road, London SW19 8LR, UK
e-mail: joe@joes-diabetes.com

K.D. Barnard and C.E. Lloyd (eds.), *Psychology and Diabetes Care*,
DOI 10.1007/978-0-85729-573-6_2,
© Springer-Verlag London Limited 2012

around this time which may explain why my diabetes occurred; I had been well up until this point and like most other 10-year-old girls. I can remember vividly my diagnosis and the subsequent weeks when adjustment was the most difficult. This chapter will explore my encounters of living with diabetes from diagnosis to treatment changes, personal experiences and feelings, and subconsciously living in fear of diabetes-related complications.

2.1.1   Diagnosis

From recollection of events leading to diagnosis, there is one day whereby it is possible to pinpoint the onset of symptoms. I had spent the day with my parents and in the afternoon went to the cinema, during which I consumed a lot of fluids and as such experienced polyuria which meant I missed the majority of the film. This day began a period of approximately two weeks whereby further symptoms presented including weight loss, reduced appetite, and lethargy.

The excessive consumption of fluids escalated to the point where I would try to hide exactly how much I was drinking as it had been noticed by members of my family, and I knew they were becoming concerned. A vivid memory I have is hiding under the dining table pretending I was playing with my toys; however, the only game I was playing was 'how much could I drink?' The weekend prior to my diagnosis, it was clear that I was very unwell; however I tried to act as 'normal' as possible and attended a party at a friend's house. My only regret is that I did not eat any sweets; as had I known what awaited me on the following Monday, I am sure I would have eaten as many as possible.

On the day of my diagnosis, I went to school as normal, however became tearful because I had a headache. My teacher was concerned as this was out of character and notified my parents. A GP appointment was made for that afternoon, and following routine tests, I was referred to the nearest hospital. It was during this time that the weight loss became worryingly apparent when the scales showed approximately four stone. My first night in hospital marked the beginning of an 8-day admission. During this time I was taught how to carry out injections independently, monitor my blood glucose levels, and educated about the adjustments necessary to my diet. At this point, I do not think I understood what 'having diabetes' fully entailed. The nurse I was in the care of on my admission had diabetes herself, something I do not think I fully benefited from; however it provided a comfort to my parents to be able to speak to someone with experience of living with the disease.

One event during my admission that I remember vividly is having a controlled hypoglycemic experience. My brother, who is 4 years my senior, and both of my parents were asked to attend the hospital ward for the day. I was asked to administer my insulin as normal but was not allowed to eat until the hypo occurred. The majority of the day was spent walking around the hospital grounds. The hypo eventually took place in the afternoon. The positive part of the experience was that I was able to discover my personal hypoglycemic symptoms with not only healthcare professionals in close proximity but also having my immediate family present so they would be able to recognize when I was hypoglycemic without being in fear of it occurring at home and know the treatment I would need. I think this experience helped me not to be in fear of hypoglycemia.

During the remainder of my admission I was allowed to spend time with my family at home on a day release basis so as to become used to returning to my 'normal' life. A part of the diagnosis experience which concerned me was returning to school and my peers finding out I was 'different'. However I had no reason to be concerned as everyone around me was very supportive. This continued throughout all of my schooling days and is still noted in present day.

The only treatment I needed at middle school was to monitor my blood glucose levels as at this time I only required insulin injections at breakfast and evening mealtimes. I can recall a time when I forgot to do this and the fear

I experienced that I would die; looking back was a little dramatic. When I reached secondary school, it was not long before I moved onto a four-a-day regimen resulting in the need to inject myself at school. The school was very support-ive and the teachers were all aware; however I remember when I initially started I would introduce myself as 'the dia-betic' in case anything ever happened during teaching.

When I was initially diagnosed I was commenced on a two-injections-a-day regimen, breakfast and evening meals; how-ever I was soon given the option to go onto a four-injections-a-day regimen allowing for more flexibility and better glycemic control, which I agreed to. Initially, the practice of injecting was met using vials of insulin and a syringe and required a specific routine in order to mix the insulins together; the preparation was the worst part of hav-ing to inject. Following this, insulin pens manually loaded with cartridges of insulin were circulated and made injecting sim-ple, and more recently disposable prefilled insulin pens have been produced removing even the need to change cartridges.

I have never missed an insulin injection mistakenly or intentionally; however I did administer my short-acting insu-lin in error one night using the dose intended for my long-acting insulin. At this point, I was still under the care of the pediatric diabetes team, and as part of the service, they pro-vided a nursing team with an out-of-hours contact. In order to overcome the problem I had to eat carbohydrate snacks regularly until the insulin action would have worn off, which lead to a fairly long and nauseous night for me and a sleepless one for my parents. Having the out-of-hours contact was a comfort for my parents while I was younger and is a service that is provided by some pediatric teams now.

I recently asked my parents what it was like for them when I was diagnosed. For my parents, their response was that of a feeling of guilt; with a potential genetic predisposition as dia-betes is prevalent on my mother's side of the family, she ini-tially blamed herself for my diagnosis. My father also had the same feelings in that it was somehow their fault and that they could have prevented the onset. My family, although protec-tive like many, tried to not be more so because of my diagnosis, and in return, I tried to be as independent as I could from the beginning to remove some of the feelings of guilt.

In the initial years I was on a fixed rate dosage of insulin, meaning each meal had to be made up of a fixed amount of carbohydrates. I found this to be one of the most restricting parts of diabetes as no matter what my appetite, I had to eat. It also posed a problem when eating out as initially, due to the type of insulin, I had to inject 30 min prior to eating and if unsure of portion sizes it often meant having to eat more than I wanted. Having such a restriction changed my relationship with food and eating; I rarely enjoyed food, it was always a case of having to eat and ensuring I ate enough carbohydrates and not about what I wanted to eat. I became quite aware of my eating patterns, especially when I had good control as at this time my mealtimes became very regimented. My daily meal plan would consist of the same cereal for breakfast, crackers and a banana for lunch, and a salad with bread for dinner. It took some time before I was able to break this cycle.

As a teenager, I did not meet the rebellion stage many teenagers experience. I was always frustrated when my control was not going well which forced me to try harder. Although strict with my diet, it was in my late teens that I found alcohol, something which I had grown up thinking was a definite 'NO'. However, my diabetes team was very supportive when I was growing up and, aware that teenagers will start to experiment with alcohol, provided education on the safest ways to do it. Many of my first experiences were on a trial and error basis; one trial being alcopops, which definitely turned out to be an error. I found that as long as I was sensible and ensured I ate prior to and post drinking alcohol I was able to maintain my blood glucose levels fairly well.

During my teenage years, I was transferred onto multiple daily injections (MDIs) using a basal bolus regimen with Lantus glargine insulin as my background (basal) and NovoRapid as my bolus which is administered at mealtimes. This insulin regimen is designed to allow freedom from restricted diet and eating patterns associated with diabetes and for many years worked very well for me.

2.1.2   Insulin Pump

The transition from a multiple daily injections regimen to continuous subcutaneous insulin infusion (CSII) pump therapy was fairly smooth. The decision, however, came over quite a long period. I was 25 years old and approximately 18 months postregistration in my nursing career. Ironically, following my appointment as a staff nurse on a diabetes specialty/acute medicine ward, my glycemic control rapidly declined. Shift work coinciding with busy and often stressful days meant it was becoming difficult to balance work with controlling my blood glucose levels. The option to transfer onto pump therapy had been broached to me prior to this, although at that point I thought that once I had settled into my new role my blood glucose levels would begin to stabilize. Unfortunately this did not happen and my decision to consider the transfer was made following a routine clinic appointment. I was due for a 12 monthly routine retinal screen, and when my consultant examined my eyes it was noted I had exudates forming in my macular in my right eye. This single event was the most frightening experience I have had over the past 16 years and I realized I had to try a different treatment option or potentially leave the career I had just began.

I met the criteria for CSII due to my HbA1c, which I believe was around the 8.5% mark. In order to fully assess my control, I was required to wear a piece of equipment known as a continuous glucose monitoring system (CGMS). This works via a subcutaneous needle and allows for the ability to assess my control over a 24-h period. I wore the monitor for a total of 7 days and was shocked by the results. It identified I was hypoglycemic at times when I did not feel symptomatic, and during night shifts my blood glucose levels fluctuated to such an extent that there was no pattern at all.

Wearing the monitor however gave me an idea of what wearing a pump continuously would be like, and it did provide me with some doubt, mainly due to size and because it felt painful whenever I made contact with the site of the needle. When I discussed this with my diabetes specialist nurse (DSN) she was very understanding and as such suggested wearing an actual pump device with saline inside before I ruled out the change in treatment completely. The CGMS monitor was larger in size, and trying out the pump, which was surprisingly comfortable, was a very beneficial experience. The body image side of wearing a pump is probably underestimated at times, and although something I did consider carefully, it turned out not to be one of my main concerns. Having diabetes to me was something I could tell people I had if I wanted to, and as I had grown very accustomed to having the disease, the lifestyle of having diabetes became almost second nature and as such I feel I have little recollection of my life prior to diagnosis. However, wearing the pump suddenly made me realize I had an illness, and that was probably the most difficult part to comprehend, rather than any actual body image concerns.

I believe body image issues related to insulin pump therapy are not gender specific; being connected to a device continuously is a huge adjustment and I feel lucky that I was able to make this change quite easily in a fairly rapid period of time. I am yet to find an outfit of clothing which is not pump friendly, something which may seem very minor but one of the main negatives people find in relation to the pump is ensuring it remains discreet, whether you are male or female.

Advances in technology have meant that some insulin pumps use Bluetooth technology via a blood glucose monitor which is used as a remote control. It allows the pump user to program and use the pump to deliver insulin doses without having to use the pump device itself directly meaning it can remain hidden under clothing. Although available to me, I am yet to utilize this as I prefer to be able to see what the pump is doing. However, I am sure it has proved to be a positive to many pump users.

When deciding to make the change to CSII from daily injections, I did discuss the option with those closest to me. Although some thought the decision was almost spontaneous as to them my control had not changed that much to make such a dramatic change at this point, my main focus was on the complications I was beginning to develop and the potential complications which could arise if I did not make any changes.

I have found the insulin pump to be revolutionary, assisting me in not only my day to day life but also with my career and being able to improve my control. I do find that I remain strict in terms of my diet, regimented to three meals a day, and still do not 'snack'; however like many people I do have my vices. Wine.

As part of the criteria for CSII, I was required to complete the DAFNE course (Dose Adjustment for Normal Eating). Carbohydrate counting is the main focus of this course with the aim to enable people with diabetes to consume food as a person without diabetes would and learn how to calculate the correct amount of insulin personally required to gain tight control. Along with this, personal correction doses are devised and education regarding exercise and how to safely consume alcohol is given. I had already completed this course prior to contemplating the pump therapy option as it is also worthwhile for patients on a basal bolus insulin regimen as carbohydrate counting and insulin dose adjustment is also beneficial for glycemic control with this regimen.

2.1.3   Positive and Negative Experiences

My healthcare experiences have always been very positive over the years, although the recent change of going onto pump therapy provided me with one of my first experiences of the emergency side of diabetes. I have a kidney defect unrelated to diabetes which increases my susceptibility to kidney infections. This has been a recurrent problem over the years; however, the first infection I had while being on the pump proved to be a different experience. The onset of urinary symptoms commenced on a Sunday. My plan was to obtain some antibiotics the following day and monitor my blood glucose levels until this time. My last blood glucose level before going to bed was 8.8 mmols; however, I underestimated how quickly blood glucose levels can increase due to infections while on pump therapy.

I awoke the following morning with a blood glucose level of approximately 17 mmols, however at this point only felt

lethargic and had loin pain. I corrected my blood glucose
level and went to work that morning as normal; however on
arrival further symptoms occurred, mainly nausea. I checked
both my ketones and blood glucose levels and was alarmed to
find that my blood glucose had reached >20 mmols, and my
ketones were >4. Although I knew this could mean I was in
my first full experience of diabetic ketoacidosis, I was more
concerned at this point to be in my nurse's uniform and having to go to the acute medical unit. Unfortunately, when
people with diabetes have an issue with their glycemic control it can often be perceived by healthcare professionals that
they have been noncompliant with their medication or their
diabetes diet and this is why problems have occurred. I was
concerned about this as the hospital I was in was not aware
of my patient background, and I did not want to be initially
perceived as being noncompliant by my colleagues. In some
ways I think I was also embarrassed as I felt as a nurse I
should have prevented this from occurring.

Following assessment, I was commenced on the treatment
for diabetic ketoacidosis almost immediately using IV insulin
on a sliding scale – a treatment I provide to patients on a
regular basis – and when I initially arrived on the ward I did
not feel particularly unwell, just extremely nauseous. With
these two components, I felt almost as if I was a nuisance and
an unfair addition to their workload. I believe added to this
was an issue of trust; having a long-term condition often
means patients will be used to taking responsibility and
charge of their own treatment, and handing this over to a
third party can be a daunting experience.

My professional experience meant that I was fully aware of
the medics management plan, the seriousness of my condition, and the need for continuous monitoring, and the medical
and nursing team kept me fully informed; it was not perceived
that I would automatically know what was happening.

I had been an inpatient in the secondary care environment a couple of years prior to this event; my first admission
in hospital since my diagnosis whereby I had to undergo a
surgical procedure for which I required anesthesia. The surgery was unrelated to my diabetes; however I required a

sliding scale for preparation which meant I was required to be admitted the day before. At this point in my career I was a student nurse and I was familiar with sliding scales from my experiences on placements. I was commenced on the IV insulin sliding scale at approximately 6:00 a.m. and knew I was on the morning list for theater. I was aware my blood glucose levels needed regular monitoring however I did not want to be seen as the 'awkward' patient and so did not challenge the medical staff when this did not happen. I checked my own blood glucose levels when I was symptomatic of hypoglycemia and was found to be hypoglycemic. I notified the nursing staff who attended to me, however the porters also arrived to take me to theater. I was very nervous as this was the first time I had received anesthesia and experienced a surgical procedure, and having hypoglycemic symptoms contributed to a fairly negative experience.

The treatment I received during my DKA (diabetic ketoacidosis) experience was exceptional; the conversion from IV insulin sliding scale back onto CSII was without fault, even though there was limited knowledge of pump therapy, it being a relatively new development. The consultant and diabetes team were fantastic; however when they had finished for the day it was quite a daunting experience. This may have been heightened, in my opinion, due to the amount of insulin I was receiving and because I did not feel in control as I was unsure of what to do. I was fairly new to insulin pump therapy treatment and it was also my first experience of being DKA, which in itself was terrifying. Having diabetes for 16 years without experience of acute emergency issues was something I was almost proud of, and I felt a degree of personal disappointment.

Although the consultant regularly contacted the department after leaving to be updated on my progress and advise me of changes to be made, I think the overall experience had frightened me into thinking I did not know how to work out the infusion rates I required and that I could make a mistake. My blood glucose levels had reduced and were within a 4–6 mmol range for the latter part of my admission;

however I still had ketones present and so required a large amount of insulin which put me at risk of hypoglycemia. I tried to take as much control over my glucose monitoring as possible, although I was concerned I would become hypoglycemic overnight and it may have been thought necessary to turn my pump off which led to a fairly sleepless night. I was discharged the following morning and the consultant was very supportive on discharge by advising me when it would be necessary to begin to reduce my insulin doses to return to my normal rates once the antibiotics had taken effect.

In one way this can be seen as a positive that patients are doing so well on CSII therapy, reducing the need for secondary care input, although as a patient it was difficult not to be frightened. I believe it identifies the need for training in all sectors of healthcare.

The entire experience was certainly a positive learning curve for me as I now know it is vital when I begin to feel unwell to increase my insulin requirements as soon as possible to prevent further complications. I believe if the event should ever occur again when I require medical input I would not have the same daunted feeling; however I think giving a third party control over my illness may always provide an unnerving experience. I do however feel much more confident with my insulin pump.

One of the initial times I experienced a kidney infection I was approximately 15 years old. I also experienced a hypoglycemic episode and I was unable to treat it independently, the first and only time this has occurred. I can remember waking and reaching for something on my bedside table, however dropping it to the floor. I have little recollection of this event, and can only retell from my mother's experience.

My mother entered my room and found me falling out of bed. I was still conscious however in a confused state and apparently spent the remainder of the time rhyming words and reciting the alphabet, at times backwards. As I had only been commenced on a course of antibiotics the previous day, my mother's initial thought was that I was having a reaction to them and took me to the nearest hospital. After taking a history, my blood glucose level was checked and I was in fact hypoglycemic. After receiving the necessary treatment I can remember becoming alert and being sat in a waiting room wearing my pyjamas and dressing gown, just what every 15 year old wants.

I can remember my mother stating the doctor was very abrupt with her when she said she had not checked my blood glucose levels; however as up until this point I had always had full hypoglycemic awareness and was rarely unwell; she reacted in the same way any mother would. However, despite having this experience of hypoglycemia, I have always been more fearful of the repercussions of hyperglycemia.

From my personal experiences of both hypoglycemia and hyperglycemia, although both dangerous, from a symptomatic perspective, hypos are often more rapidly treated, thus the symptoms have a shorter duration than the correction process involved in hyperglycemia. There have been situations when I have tried to hide the symptoms and treat hypos as discreetly as possible so as not to concern the people I am with and because there is an element of embarrassment. Many people with diabetes have their own individual symptoms which they relate to hypoglycemia. My own consist of a general feeling of lethargy, headaches, and visible tremors. If nocturnal I have been known to wake feeling very hot and clammy, a part of diabetes which used to concern me about staying with friends due to an embarrassment element. However, all of my friends are aware of my diabetes and also educated to a point of what they need to do if I am ever unwell and unable to treat myself. I am very lucky to have the support network I have around me.

I often wonder about the type of person I would be if I did not have diabetes. From diagnosis I have tried to be as independent as possible with my treatment and overall management of my illness. I am quite controlling of my illness although try not to dwell on being diagnosed as I have always been of the mindset that there is little I can change. I approach general life in a fairly laid-back and relaxed manner, although

I wonder if I may be more carefree and spontaneous, something that is not possible at present, unless I have all of my pump equipment with me! It is necessary to carry spare consumables with you at all times: spare cannulae, infusion sets, batteries, fillable syringes for insulin, to name just a few. However, the only change this has made to my general life from previously having only glucose monitoring equipment and insulin pens is that I require a bigger bag!

2.1.4   Stress

A side of diabetes which I have found to be frustrating is the impact stress has on glycemic control. While on multiple daily injections, events occurred within my family which lead to a fairly stressful period of time. This can be related to my HbA1c, which increased substantially, and my daily blood glucose levels which were often erratic and required correction doses at nearly every mealtime. However, due to my age the connection to psychological changes was not made by myself or my diabetes team as they were unaware of my personal changes and as this was also when puberty occurred it was difficult to know which was the main contributor.

More recently, however, I have had dramatic relationship changes within my personal life, occurring since my commencement on insulin pump therapy. Initially, I obtained fairly good control quickly; however this soon declined and it has been difficult to assess how much insulin I have required, resulting in erratic blood glucose levels at times. Due to my emotional status during this time, it was very difficult as it was not only necessary to deal with general life problems, it also means you have to focus on your diabetes control. It was difficult to deal with the emotional problems when my control had to take precedence at times, however, I soon realized until I faced the problems in my personal life, I was not going to improve any part of my control. This did lead to a period where I did not feel in control of anything which was very difficult and my glycemic control was dealt with on a day to day basis, whereby correction doses had to be used far too often rather than looking at my control on a grand scale. During my episode of diabetic ketoacidosis, when discussing with the diabetes specialist nursing team about recent life events, it was suggested that this may have contributed to its occurrence, having raised glucose levels due to stress coinciding with my existing kidney defect may have multiplied my infection susceptibility. This highlighted to me how important it is to face problems in my personal life. Now I feel more settled, my control has once again improved and I am hoping it continues to do so and I will once again feel the full benefits of insulin pump therapy.

***

2.2   Joe Fraser

2.2.1   Living with Type 1 Diabetes

Being diagnosed with type 1 diabetes was a big shock for me; there was no genetic link, and it really just came out of the blue. I was 13 and in the car with my family going to Paris for a relative's wedding. It was an early morning, and I was asleep until I woke up when we were on the motorway in France, really needing to pee. I also had this strange thirst, a kind of salt-sweet taste in my mouth that the Fanta I was drinking was doing very little to get rid of. We could not stop quickly as it was incredibly foggy, and by the time we reached a service station it felt like I had bruised my bladder with holding it in!

We eventually got to Paris and went to the wedding. I felt basically fine, if a little jaded from an early morning and long car trip, and a bit disturbed by the intense need to pee I had had. The rest of the weekend went well, and we picked up a load of lovely food from a hypermarket on the way home.

I was feeling pretty tired and run-down on the Monday after the trip and took the day off school. I felt better the next day though, went in, and essentially everything was normal. However, I was strangely tired when I got home and decided to treat myself by gorging on some of the wonderful food and drink we had brought back. That night I woke up between six and eight times to pee. Something was definitely wrong. I went to the GP the next day, had a glucose test (which was 33 mmol/l!), was formally diagnosed at hospital, and had my first insulin injection that night.

I struggle to remember my thoughts or feelings accurately at this particular time. I think there simply was not time to register any real response, particularly because I could not really tell how serious the situation was. A classmate of mine had been diagnosed with type 1 diabetes a few months beforehand, but he seemed OK with it. With hindsight, I was incredibly lucky with the speed of my diagnosis (from presenting initial symptoms to taking my first injection took less than a week), but at the time, I think that contributed to my later sense of alienation. I think that if I had, a more obvious period of illness perhaps the transition to treating myself would have seemed more logical and progressive, rather than an abrupt change that I suddenly had to make.

Soon after diagnosis I decided that my diabetes must be my responsibility foremost if not solely mine. This assertiveness was precipitated by at least three main factors. The first was purely practical: people would not be around to look after me all the time, so I had better get a pretty good handle on how everything worked. Secondly, I did not want people to feel that they did have to look after me at all – I was even fairly keen to forgo any kind of medical checkups. This was my problem, and I would deal with it. I think this is as close to teenage 'rebellion' I ever got with diabetes (!), mainly because the risks of not treating the disease with its proper respect seemed not worth contemplating. Finally, in a world that had turned completely on its head, taking responsibility for the diabetes, making it my job, was the only option open to me to regain some sense of control.

I did not find having diabetes easy to begin with. Perhaps, I did not help myself with how I managed my diabetes; there is a fine line between independence and isolation which I crossed during this time. I am not sure that anyone does think "brilliant," but I felt very low and vulnerable at the time. It was a big shock. The problem was not even with measuring and injecting, directly. Yes, they were a bit painful, and they seemed fairly constant (as if they were the main thing you did with your day), but it was what they represented that I had particular difficulty with. I was used to eating what I liked, when I liked, and suddenly that freedom was taken away from me. I think there was also a feeling of being betrayed by my body. "How could you do this to me? What have I done to deserve this?" Alongside that was a realization that diabetes was not that bad: some relatively painful measuring on the fingers and a couple of injections a day meant that I was alive. It could have been worse; I could have been born before 1921 or had cancer, or liver failure, or kidney problems. Those comparisons did not really help though – the point was I had this problem that meant I had to change the way I lived in order to treat it.

Change of that kind is not easy, especially when you are trying to learn how everything works, and the tools you are given to treat your problem do not help you. Two injections a day is, in my humble opinion, a really clumsy system of control and does not give you the scope to learn quickly from mistakes. I do not remember having any massive hypos or hypers in the early days, but getting a glucose result that was on target was definitely more down to fluke, than brilliant management, or exceptional self-control. Waking up was a real bore: first thing, stab your finger; measure and tediously write down the fairly random result; then inject some insulin. The system of twice-daily injections also means you have to eat snacks between meals, and allied to the contemporary clinical advice to basically "eat carbohydrates"; I put on quite a lot of weight. This inability to regulate my eating did not do wonders for my self-esteem. I see now that there was a whole complex array of psychological problems interacting: a shock and sudden feeling of vulnerability, being compounded by an inability to take control causing a sense of inadequacy (itself a heightening of the thought that your body had failed you), all being exacerbated by my increasing weight. The real problem with getting fatter was what it represented. Though I had never been particularly thin, the fat became the most obvious sign of the change that had occurred to me, and my own inability to take control and come to terms with it.

In many ways, putting on weight was helped by my general inactivity after diagnosis: I took a lot of time off school that year. Mostly, it was because I felt genuinely bad. I had chronic sinusitis, which definitely does not lift your mood. A few times though, I just did not want to go in, particularly as no one seemed to be sympathetic to what had happened to me. I think people at school thought I was just being lazy all the time and I definitely remember being taken aside by a sports teacher to check that my absences from his lessons tallied with my actual days away. That attitude did not encourage my regular attendance (!) and was a concrete example of the conflict taking place: everything for everyone else at school was normal, but for me the entire world had changed. I did not want to lose touch with my friends, but I also could not stand to be around them. The outside world was too different from my own inner one. I felt alienated and out of control.

It is from this period of my life that I take my understanding of diabetic stigma. It is a general sense of inadequacy, laced with guilt, and shot through with loneliness. I do not remember anyone ever saying "you cannot" do anything because of your diabetes to me, but there seemed to be a part of the world that was closed off from me now that I had diabetes. Guilt works its way into this emotion because you (as the one with diabetes, the person nominally in charge) have let down your future self (by storing up potential complications) and those you care about. You then become lonely because these are emotions that as a teenager (a) you cannot often articulate and (b) would not want to express even if you could and (c) you have no one that can understand these feelings readily at hand.

2.2.2   Taking Control

The second year was far better than the first. I was getting used to the tedium of measuring and injecting by now and found it less of a burden: they no longer dominated my days. I had also started doing some exercise over the summer, so by the time it was autumn I was thinner, if not thin, and was feeling more in control. I still was not well all the time but I could deal with it better, having had the experience of the year before. Since I was at school more, I saw my friends more, and began to go out, drink a little, and meet girls. Life was better!

Now that I look back on it, I was still adjusting to having diabetes during that second year. The first year was simply taken up with the "shock and awe" of diagnosis. It was during the second year that my independent approach began to pay dividends, as I was confident enough to go out and meet people. The second year was when I realized that my diabetes was not going to go away – that the nightmare of the first year could repeat itself unless I took charge. And it was also at this time that I had enough distance to look back on the year before and try to work out how it had affected me. I do not remember having any moments of clarity or any great insights, but I think it was another sign of my increasing confidence with diabetes, and a symptom of my desire to understand it and take control.

It was only in my third year that I began to really take charge though when I began to do a lot of running. I managed to lose the rest of the weight that I had put on when first diagnosed with diabetes by matching up the amount of running I was doing to the insulin I was taking. I kept playing around with my diabetes: seeing how much I would need to run to bring my glucose level back to normal, having 'boosted' it by not taking quite enough insulin or eating more than I needed. I was not right all the time by any means, but I was feeling more in control. And when things went well, when I could match up the concrete sensation of exercise to the rather abstract numbers on a glucose meter, I got an amazing sense of understanding and empowerment.

My feeling of achievement was only helped when I started on the four-a-day injection system after taking some exams when I turned sixteen. While there were some small teething problems to begin with – the odd big hypo here and there as I found the right balance of things – I loved the four-a-day system. The brilliant thing about this system is its directness, and the ability to correct doses accurately. Instead of the broad-brush strokes of the two-a-day, where you can never really be sure how the various factors affect you, on four-a-day, you can work out on a gram by gram basis how much, say, a pack of crisps chips will raise your blood sugar. It meant I could start to get a handle on the mechanics of the disease and feel confident and flexible enough to do anything. However, with that flexibility I learnt that still the best way to stay in control was to stick fairly closely to a routine which you could then adjust to any situation (with a significant amount of educated guess work).

This is not to say that flexibility is not without its price – no matter what I do there is a little voice inside asking, "How is this going to affect your blood sugar?" It is the result of the need to be conscious of your body, aware of its mechanisms and how these will be affected by numerous factors, and, with that information, be able to manage everything so that your blood sugar remains within safe limits. It is perhaps not surprising that, particularly to begin with, things do go wrong and that the whole process is fairly tiring. I suppose the closest analogy I can give is that learning to be 'diabetic' is like learning to drive a manual car – you make mistakes and can become fatigued by the need to concentrate all the time. Eventually though my blood sugar regulation became almost unconscious, like changing gear. The tricky thing is that each person is like a different car, on a different road, in different conditions. Only you, as the driver, know which gear feels right at any moment, or as the person with diabetes, how much insulin to take.

It is perhaps a slightly strange way to be, but I tend to think of my body in mechanical terms. I constantly think of factors that can affect me in terms of the amount they will raise my blood sugar and over what period of time. There is no quick trick to working this out – it is purely a case of trying to isolate other factors and experimenting through trial and error until you find out that, say, in hot weather you should reduce your background insulin by one or two units even if you are not that active. Even then, all you have really done is work out the ballpark figure; the trick is to then finesse your dose so that it works within the constraints of what you actually want to do with a day. If you are just doing one particular thing that can be accounted for but if a few different activities emerge during a day, it can still be quite tricky to handle.

2.2.3   10% of the Time…

Even if I am fairly happy and feel on top of my diabetes it is pretty tough to remain in perfect control. There are so many different factors to think about that, sooner or later, I am bound to make a mistake and end up too high or too low. Being hyper- or hypoglycemic can make me feel pretty down-hearted, particularly if both or either happens consistently. Illness can be particularly frustrating; I feel horrible and my sugars keep rising (making me feel worse) unless I make fairly dramatic changes to my insulin doses. On one level, there is the actual physical sensation of each of the conditions. Not all people with diabetes say they can feel when they are hyperglycemic, but a significant number (myself included) can. I feel tired and groggy, need to pee, and have an unpleasant thirst. It is not terrible but neither is it fun. Going hypo is completely different. Whereas hyperglycemia can make me feel lethargic, hypoglycemia (in its mild state – in its severe state I become unconscious) gives me masses of nervous energy – but only to get food! It is a hard sensation to describe, but I feel weak to my core, desperately greedy, and somewhat indulgent. When I was diagnosed it was definitely taught that I should not have chocolate and sweets, so whenever I had a hypo I would use it as an excuse to gorge, which would then usually shoot my sugars up afterward. This set up a fairly strange relationship with hypos – I would not induce them (as they really are not much fun), but I would not hate them either. I guess they gave me a break from the norm of trying to be in control all the time.

Perhaps my thinking on hypers and hypos is slightly skewed because I am lucky not to have had an extreme hypo (when you go into a coma) and only one DKA (though that was one too many), but I do not think the physical symptoms are that awful. It is really the psychological effect of both extremes of glucose that are the problem. They remind me of my sense of 'difference' and, ultimately, of my lack of control. They are the 'face' of diabetes' effects on the patient, enforcing a disassociation between the managing mind and the managed body. The effect is to make me very conscious of how things are affecting or may affect me.

This self-consciousness is vital to me as a person with diabetes: I need to be able to estimate what my blood sugar is doing to feel comfortable doing just about anything. I become prepared; I plan for possibilities because if I do not, there is a significant chance things will go wrong. Say I am out walking and I start to go hypo but do not have anything sweet on me, or money to buy anything, or there are not any shops nearby – what will happen? I go hypo, possibly slip into a coma, cause myself, my friends, and family a load of grief, put an unnecessary strain on the health system, and lose my dignity. I guess the last point is one of the most important. Most people are self-conscious to a certain extent – they dress or behave in a certain way that is appropriate to their surroundings, and if they misjudge this, they can feel awkward. With people with diabetes, it is the same but more extreme. There is a sense of betraying the trust to look after yourself that is given to you by the emotional and medical authorities of your life.

It sounds strange that you would need a reminder of diabetes' seriousness considering the complications that can arise from poor control – retinopathy, nephropathy, amputations, etc but once you are quite well-controlled and used to a routine, having diabetes just feels normal. That is the stage I was at just before I finished university. I went to Oxford and, in spite of stressful essay crises and the occasional boozy binge, I was in good shape. Having got through just over two and half years of working almost as hard as I could, I had about a week off from finishing my last piece of coursework, before having to start revision with 6 weeks to go until the first exam. I was under a ton of pressure for the length of this period with a strict routine of early mornings (for a student), no alcohol, daily exercise, and working to midnight or beyond. This was then followed by over a week of exams and constant work outside of the exam hall.

By the time the last exam was over, I was absolutely exhausted although very happy that it was all over. I walked back to college with the rest of the English students, and we began to celebrate.

The trouble was that I was completely unused to drinking after 6 weeks' abstinence and shattered by working as hard as possible; I got drunk very quickly indeed! I had managed to eat a bit of lunch but I was so drunk that I had not taken any insulin. After weaving in and out of consciousness over the next 20 hours, being sick, and so confused I thought it best not to take any insulin, I eventually worked out that something was not right and admitted myself to hospital. It was quite a shock. It never occurred to me to change the way I was living or managing my diabetes. I suppose this is one of the 'psychological complications' of diabetes – in my view it makes you tougher. Not only do you have to come through a big shock upon diagnosis, but you also have to steel yourself (quite literally) every day to accept the demands of the disease.

From my point of view, 'being diabetic' is simply my lifestyle – I do experience some frustrations about not achieving the ideal control that I aspire to, but not performing at your very best 100% of the time is a normal aspect of living no matter what you do.

Chapter 3
Supporting Resilience and Positive Outcomes in Families, Children, and Adolescents

Deborah Christie and Katharine D. Barnard

3.1 Introduction

Grasping the immediate and long-term implications of diagnosis of diabetes is a complex process for the child or young person as well as their parents and the wider family. Learning to live with diabetes is the beginning of a long and challenging journey. At a practical level, it will involve regular visits to hospital, a need to "adhere" to complex medical regimens, and will demand changes in food and activities. Immediate and ongoing medical investigations may be invasive, uncomfortable, or painful with ongoing treatment regimens

D. Christie (✉)
Child and Adolescent Psychological Services,
University College London Hospitals NHS Foundation Trust,
250 Euston Rd, London NW1 2PQ, UK
e-mail: deborah.christie@uclh.nhs.uk

K.D. Barnard
Faculty of Medicine, University of Southampton,
Enterprise Road, Southampton Science Park, Chilworth,
Southampton, SO16 7NS, UK
e-mail: k.barnard@soton.ac.uk

K.D. Barnard and C.E. Lloyd (eds.), *Psychology and Diabetes Care*,
DOI 10.1007/978-0-85729-573-6_3,
© Springer-Verlag London Limited 2012

47

requiring medication, injections, blood measurements, and brain or body scans. Taking in the immediate demands of treatment can be confusing and frustrating. The realization of the potential long-term impact of the illness on a young person's hopes, dreams, and ambitions can be devastating.

> **Vignette**
> Mark aged 10 was admitted to the pediatric ward with diabetic ketoacidosis. The family was told that he had diabetes and would need to have injections every day. Mark became distressed every time the nurses tried to give him his insulin injections. His mum appeared overwhelmed by all of the information that she was given by the team. Mark's dad was unable to come to the hospital because he was looking after Mark's younger brother and sister. At the weekend, Mark told one of the nurses that he thought he was never going to be able to be a professional footballer because of the diabetes. He also said that he did not want anyone at school to know about the diabetes as no one would like him if he had needles in the classroom.

Mark and his mum met with the diabetes clinical nurse specialist who explained about the different kinds of pens that he could use. Mark spent some time with the ward activity coordinator and decided that being able to do the injections would make his friends think he was really brave. The diabetes nurse arranged to come into his school and help him tell his friends about diabetes. She gave him a magazine that had stories from famous people including Olympic athletes and footballers to reassure him that diabetes would not stop him doing anything that he wanted to do.

Lazarus and Folkman [1] suggested that people initially appraise whether a life event is harmful, beneficial, or benign. This is followed by a secondary appraisal which considers whether the "event" can be overcome to either minimize the negative consequences or optimize adaptation. Coping involves implementing strategies that involve assessing what we think about the event and then to consider what we do about it [1]. The way that children, young people, and families appraise this threat influences their ability to cope with the situation [2].

The role of the pediatric diabetes team is to empower children, young people with diabetes, and their families to adopt positive adjustment strategies. Positive adjustment is thought of in normative developmental terms as positive emotional well-being, age appropriate behavior, and developmentally appropriate self-esteem/self-worth.

Following the initial diagnosis, families go through a period of limbo beginning with uncertainty and worry and then slowly transition into a "new normal" by reconstructing their world. Parents and young people are often angry at the initial diagnosis. They can be angry with each other for "causing the illness" by passing on "bad genes" or not having gone to the doctors early enough. Children can often be angry at parents for not having protected them. Young children often have "magical thinking" where they believe that certain events or thoughts have caused something to happen. Siblings can sometimes think they caused the diabetes to happen by saying something nasty or children can believe their parents "gave them" the diabetes during a visit to hospital.

Susan was 5 years and had been diagnosed with diabetes 6 months earlier. Susan rarely spoke to the nurses in the consultations. Her mum said that Susan would not give her cuddles anymore and had started being very difficult when she was supposed to have her injections. Susan was better behaved with dad. Susan and her parents agreed to meet with the team psychologist who talked to Susan and her parents about what had happened to her when she came into hospital 6 months ago. Susan told the psychologist that she was angry with her mummy for taking her to hospital and giving her diabetes when they were there.

The psychologist asked the diabetes nurse specialist to meet with her Susan and her parents. They used a story about a family of bears where the little bear gets diabetes to help Susan understand about what happens when you get diabetes and where it comes from. In the story, the mummy and daddy bear helped the little bear understand how insulin is a medicine you need to take every day so that you can stay well and have fun. Susan enjoyed these sessions and her parents reported significant improvements in her behavior.

Grief is also reported in relation to loss of how life used to be, as well as a loss of spontaneity with restrictions on activities may create a sense that things will never be the same again [3]. Children and young people are unable to leave their house or visit friends without having to remember hypo equipment and their glucose meter and insulin. They will have to learn to think about carbohydrate content every time they eat a meal or a snack instead of just eating it and enjoying it. Over a course of 24 h, a child, young person, or parent will need to "think" about a diabetes-related behavior up to 33 times if they are following a multiple injection regimen.

It is important that healthcare professionals understand the need to give families, children, and young people a chance to discuss and explore these feelings in a safe, nonjudgmental environment with a member of the team they trust. Some families find it helpful to meet with a member of the psychology team; however for others the suggestion that they go and see the "psychological person" makes them feel like their reaction to the diagnosis and management of diabetes is abnormal, that they are perceived as "not coping," and therefore any referral suggestion is resented and/or rejected. Providing emotional support is not restricted to psychologists, however, with each team member being able to practice reflective listening and provide emotional support, offering families a chance to talk about how they are feeling in an open and honest way without fear of retribution or being told what they need to "do."

Practice Tips
- All members of the team should be able to offer reassurance that feelings are personal and "OK" and explore these feelings with families to help them resolve their ambiguities.
- Platitudes such as "it will get better in time" or "it will get better soon" should be avoided as they often come across as patronizing, and in truth, diabetes will never get better; the only thing that will change is how families adapt and support self-management.

Our experience is that a solution-focused approach fits with models of empowerment that are seen as increasingly relevant in the management of long-term chronic illness. The approach offers teams and families a collaborative way of thinking about difficulties with injections, finger pricks, managing eating difficulties, how diabetes gets in the way of family communication, and the effect of sadness or anger associated with living with diabetes.

The starting point for this approach is to engage children and families in a conversation which invites the family to focus on resources rather than deficits. It highlights areas that can be drawn on later in the conversation and sets the scene for positive change [4]. We begin by identifying examples of strengths, abilities, and resources. Parents are asked to describe strengths and abilities they are proud of in their son or daughter.

Box 3.1: Identifying Strengths and Abilities
What do you enjoy at school?
What is your favorite lesson/subject?
What do you like doing when you are not at school?
What else are you good at?

3.2   Impact of Diabetes

Diabetes can have a substantial impact on emotional life, lifestyle, education, self-esteem, and social relationships, as well as physical well-being in comparison to healthy peers [5]. Diagnosis during adolescence can both prevent the development of independence as well as impact on independence that has already been successfully achieved [6]. When families start to build a new world that incorporates the illness, they make physical and emotional adaptations and constantly revise their assumptions of the world. Lowes et al. [7] found that for families living with diabetes, the longer the time after diagnosis, the better the adjustment to "normal" life. However, the parents were clear that they never fully "accepted" the diagnosis. Although they adjust to the management of the diabetes, they still described episodes of grief 7 years post diagnosis. This reaction was triggered by changes in regimen, injections, hospitalization, discussions about diabetes control, worry about complications, attending clinics, and meeting new medical teams – anything that reminded them that their child is different [8]. Cadman described how parents of children with a chronic illness experience poorer marital satisfaction with mothers at greater risk of negative mood [9].

3.2.1   Emotional Well-Being

Although preexisting genetic risk factors may contribute to the development of depression, environmental factors such as family functioning alongside the potential burden of diabetes over time may exacerbate the development of depressive symptoms in children and young people with diabetes [10, 11]. In addition, the parents of young children with type 1 diabetes experience depression and depressive symptomatology as a consequence of the additional caring burden associated with type 1 diabetes. In a recent systematic review of parental fear of hypoglycemia, parents reported feelings of despair, isolation, and fear, and in extreme cases had considered suicide as the burden of caring for their child with diabetes had become too much to cope with [12].

The multidisciplinary diabetes teams in partnership with families are ideally placed to attend to changes in mood or behaviors in children and adolescents. Changes in metabolic control, an increase in canceled appointments, or failure to attend appointments may signal emerging emotional difficulties associated with problems living with diabetes. An increase in hospital admissions should trigger an assessment of potential psychological distress that may be connected with difficulty administering insulin or be due to deliberate over or under administration [13].

Insulin omission is the most common purging method in individuals with diabetes and an eating disorder, with as many as 31% of young females with type 1 diabetes acknowledging having previously reduced their insulin to promote weight loss [14]. Insulin omission has been reported to increase throughout the teenage years [15], occurring at the sensitive developmental stage in which responsibility for diabetes care is increasingly delegated from parent to child with supervision of self-care decreasing. Peveler et al. [15] suggest that as many as 25% of young females with type 1 diabetes may develop clinically important disturbances of eating habits and attitudes at some point in their lives.

The diagnosis of a medical condition and its associated treatment regimen can also cause prominent anxiety symptoms. It is important to separate general childhood anxieties from diabetes-specific anxieties. The "additional burden of diabetes" creates significant challenges for children, young people, and their families. There are many general diabetes anxieties such as wanting to maintain good control to avoid the threat of complications, or anxiety around injecting at school, or how young people feel they are perceived by others, etc.

Generalized or specific anxiety disorders that may have existed before the onset of diabetes, disease-related anxiety as well as treatment-related anxiety have all been identified as having a negative impact on metabolic outcome and subsequent quality of life of children, young people, and families [16].

Fear of needles and injections is a common specific phobia significantly exacerbated by a diagnosis of diabetes. Fear of needles can result in high levels of avoidance behavior and a refusal to give insulin injections or complete blood tests [17]. The anxiety is often extreme and easily observed, especially in younger children, where there is loud and obvious protest. In older children and adolescents, anxiety about needles may only become apparent through increasingly poor metabolic control, high blood glucose measurements, or a failure to regularly monitor blood glucose.

Practice Tip
Make sure to check with parents in case they are anxious about needles. This can often be transmitted to children without realizing. Early identification of needle worry can be helped by a referral to a play therapist or activity coordinators. If the worry does not resolve quickly using play and/or behavioral techniques, a clinical psychologist can offer a more structured approach to managing the anxiety. The longer worry about needles is left, the harder it can be to treat.

3.2.2   Problems at School

School can be a significant challenge with the need for injections, blood glucose testing, and immediate response to high or low blood glucose causing disruption in the classroom. Twenty-four studies were included in the meta-analysis carried out by Naguib et al. [18]. They found a significant impact on sustained attention, visuospatial ability, motor speed, writing, and reading. Consistent with Gaudieri et al. [19], children with diabetes also showed a reduction in verbal and performance IQ. While these reductions are small, they place children at a disadvantage in relation to peers, especially in demanding academic environments. Nonverbal intellectual abilities are particularly vulnerable to the effects of early onset diabetes. Naguib et al.

suggested that this is probably accounted for by the vulnerability of perceptual skills to early childhood brain insult [20] and the greater impact of diffuse diabetes-related metabolic changes on the young brain [21, 22]. It has been suggested that reduced motor speed may be the childhood equivalent of the slowing of mental ability found in adult studies [23]. The visuospatial anomalies, reduced motor speed, and sustained attention effects may underpin subsequent difficulties with reading and writing. Severe hypoglycemic attacks were also found to be associated with small but significant effects on short-term verbal memory.

Hospital appointments can impact on attendance, performance, motivation, and attitude toward school as well as causing children/young people to miss out on recreational and sporting activities [24]. Children struggle to catch up on work which impacts upon exam results and future career choice. Young people interviewed about the impact of a chronic illness on school describe how missing school can cause relationship problems. Such as difficulty in reinitiating friendships on return to school as well as struggling to handle questions about their absence and illness [3].

If problems at school are suspected it may be helpful to suggest a neuropsychological assessment to determine any relationship with possible cognitive impairments described in the research. The results of this assessment can also provide practical information to help improve management of children and young people with T1DM.

3.2.3 Family Factors That Influence Adjustment

Family cohesion is a key mediator of childhood temperament, personality, and emotionality as well as temperament, competence, self motivation, and problem-solving skills. Family cohesion, parenting satisfaction, socioeconomic resources, maternal employment, social support, and parental education are all related to positive psychological adjustment in children with diabetes [3]. Low levels of family conflict, good family relations and support, marital satisfaction, and a social support network lead to good adjustment [24]. Soliday et al. [25] reported that irrespective of whether a child was chronically ill or not, families with higher cohesion and expressiveness and less conflict had less parental stress.

The amount of stress reported by children and families is related to the ability to manage the medical regimen as well as the frequency of hospital visits [26]. Diabetes-related stress (e.g., carbohydrate counting, difficulty with injections, and blood testing) mediates between metabolic control and adjustment and influences quality of life and well-being [3].

Research has demonstrated that a substantial proportion of individuals who do not report depressive symptoms still feel unable to cope with their diabetes. It has been suggested that these people are experiencing diabetes-related distress or are "burned out" by their diabetes. Diabetes burnout occurs when a person feels "overwhelmed by diabetes and by the frustrating burden of diabetes self-care" [14].

Diabetes-specific family conflict is often associated with high levels of diabetes-related distress [27]. These emotions may be very different to feelings of depression; however, they can still be very destructive and have serious implications for care [28].

Maria was 14 years of age and had been excluded from school for aggressive behavior. She was admitted to hospital five times over 6 months in DKA, three of which required admission to ITU. Maria and her mother had an explanation for each event and felt that the team was critical and bullying. Maria denied omitting insulin or doing anything that contributed to the poor control. During a 4-week admission Maria refused to go to school while she was on the ward. She denied low mood or any other symptoms of depression. She told the team that she felt blamed and that she was being picked on. She said that she hated diabetes and thought that trying to do four or more blood tests every day was "stupid" and that she just wanted to get on with her life. She refused to meet with the psychologist and only agreed to come to clinic when a referral to social services was finally made.

The psychologist joined the family and the doctor at the next clinic appointment and explained how her job was not to work with people who were mad but that she met with people to help them think about how to make diabetes less of a monster and a bully. She positively connoted Maria's desire to get on with her life and how it must feel like everyone was on her back. She wondered if she and Maria were to meet a couple of times to think about how to sort this out, it might make people less worried about her and would help to get people off her back. Maria agreed to meet for an initial consultation the following month and decided that she would carry on coming every time she came to clinic.

Parental fear of hypoglycemia, anxiety, and depression are also reported to be common [12]. Parents have a number of diabetes-specific worries and anxieties that include fear of hypoglycemia and associated seizures both during the day and at night, anxiety associated with frequent blood glucose monitoring, fear of "not being there" despite daily management being relentless, and fear that others, such as babysitters, teachers, and others will be unable to provide appropriate care for their child. Experiencing hypoglycemia at some point in time after diagnosis and engaging in subsequent avoidance behaviors contribute to the problem. Some parents report that they will run blood glucose levels "slightly" higher than recommended to avoid acute episodes of hypoglycemia [12]. The knock-on effect of this will be a higher HbA1c. Paradoxically, chronically higher HbA1c levels are associated with the signs of acute hypoglycemia presenting at higher blood glucose levels, i.e., rather than 3.9 and below. This means hypoglycemic signs can be present when the patient is actually hyperglycemic and not hypoglycemic. Thus, parents engage in further avoidance behaviors, leading to even higher HbA1c, causing a spiraling effect of worsening diabetes control. With every 1% increase in HbA1c, there is an associated 60% increase in risk of long-term complications. This behavior can be either conscious or subconscious with fear a strong motivating factor to maintain such maladaptive coping despite the long-term risks.

A recent literature review of the contributing factors to parental fear reported that mothers of young children with type 1 diabetes reported greater fear of hypoglycemia and took more steps to avoid it than fathers did. Mothers and fathers reported the same level of worry about hypoglycemia though. Fathers, however, experience greater levels of parenting stress and have lower confidence in their ability to manage their child's diabetes, reporting greater anxiety and increased hopelessness than mothers. Half of parents reported the child experiencing an episode of hypoglycemia three to five times per week [29]. However, the severity of hypoglycemia seems more important in causing fear than frequency, especially in parents whose child had experienced a hypoglycemic seizure. Almost a third of children with diabetes (32%) had experienced at least one hypoglycemia seizure during their lifetime [30]. It is perhaps unsurprising that parents of children who had experienced a hypoglycemic seizure within the past year had significantly greater overall fear of hypoglycemia (both in terms of avoidance behavior and the extent to which they worry about it) than those whose children had not experienced a seizure. Mothers whose children had a history of passing out experienced far greater worry than mothers whose children had never lost consciousness. Furthermore, children who had experienced a seizure with loss of consciousness had a significantly higher percentage of self-monitoring of blood glucose (SMBG) values above the desired target range than young children with no history of seizures, which suggests that parents of these children are indeed allowing higher than desired blood glucose levels to avoid hypoglycemia.

Increased maternal depression and anxiety are associated with greater fear of hypoglycemia [31], with maternal symptoms of anxiety and depression unrelated to their child's metabolic control. Although surprisingly, in most children their HbA1c was below the treatment goals recommended for their age group (average HbA1c 6.86%). "Not being there" if the child needs them is a major cause of anxiety for many parents as well as them having a hypo during the night and consequently not waking up in the morning.

Siblings can also struggle with the diagnosis and may experience guilt that they remain healthy; however they also often feel excluded and describe missing out on parental attention [24].

Stephen was the 9-year-old brother of 7-year-old James who had been diagnosed with diabetes 2 years ago. Stephen started struggling at school and became increasingly withdrawn at home. During one of the visits to the clinic, Stephen told the nurse that he felt sad and wished that he had diabetes like James.

The family met with the psychologist that worked with the diabetes team. She asked Stephen and James to tell her when diabetes had come into their house and where it lived. She asked the boys to draw a picture of what diabetes looked like and who it picked on. She asked James to tell her what sort of things were good about diabetes and what were the not so good things. She asked him to tell her what things Stephen did that helped James keep diabetes in its place. She talked to Stephen about how he learned to become such a help to James and how come he was able to do these things. Mum and dad were invited to talk about Stephen's positive skills and abilities and if this was something that they had taught him or whether he was just naturally good at being helpful. The psychologist explained to Stephen that there was a special society for brothers that helped younger brothers who had diabetes and asked if was willing to be nominated for an award. Stephen readily agreed to this and said he would be happy to come back in a month and talk about all the ways he and James had found to keep diabetes in its place so that the team could help other little boys.

Practice Tips
- Make sure to check with families what is going well and identify the skills abilities and resources that are making this possible.
- Early identification of difficulties can often be addressed relatively easily before they develop into a more complex situation.
- Always give families an opportunity to talk about concerns and try to think how to address them using available resources.
- Reassure parents, children, and young people that they are not the only ones to have these difficulties. Normalizing the concerns can often be very reassuring.

3.2.4 Positive Coping Strategies

Families use a range of different strategies to cope at different times in the course of the illness. Planful problem solving is one of the most adaptive strategies using positive reappraisal which involves taking positive steps when thinking about the impact of the illness. Positive appraisal can help replace anger and sadness with satisfaction and pride. Engaging and searching for help and advice and social support are other positive and adaptive coping strategies used by families [32]. Parental stress is also reduced by having good information and having the opportunity to speak to other parents in a similar situation [33]. Access to information has been significantly improved by the development of the internet, although families may often need help negotiating the good, the bad, and the ugly that increasingly exists in "the cloud."

The diabetes team can model and encourage planful problem solving during clinic visits, also creating opportunities for families to contact each other as well as pointing families in the direction of positive supportive literature and websites.

Coping strategies that involve distancing, escape, and avoidance are more likely to be used when high levels of stress are experienced by parents [26]. Mutual support between the child and parent, anticipatory coping, and social comparison are positive coping strategies used by children with chronic illness [3]. If mother and child feel that each are uninvolved, there is a greater incidence of depression and negative mood. A collaborative partnership between parent and child provides a buffer for negative emotions with fewer depressive symptoms and more positive mood – particularly for adolescents [34].

Children worry about what their future holds, but where there was parental involvement they were found to be more optimistic about the future [35]. In one study, self-esteem was increased when children went away to educational and special event days [3]. Diabetes summer camps offering sports and recreational activities alongside daily diabetes self-management training also show short-term changes in self-management and knowledge, however have failed to demonstrate lasting improvements in HbAlc levels without ongoing support [36, 37].

John was 13 years old and had lived with diabetes for 4 years. Since transferring to secondary school, his parents were trying to get him to take more control over his diabetes self-management. John was able to do his injections without being reminded; however, he would always forget blood testing and would get into arguments with his mother when she reminded him to check his blood glucose. John had never met anyone else with diabetes, however agreed to go on a diabetes camp. John spent a week with other young people with diabetes. He came back from camp and started doing regular blood tests.

3.3   Treatment Approaches

Few interventions have been trialed with younger children. Northam et al. [38] pointed out that most studies have used diabetes-specific unstandardized interventions in groups of adolescents. There are few studies targeting a specific psychological disorder such as behavior problems or depression, both of which are known to be increased in children with diabetes and for which effective standardized interventions are available. Recently Snoek et al. [39] showed that a cognitive behavioral therapy group (CBT) decreased depressive symptoms for up to 12 months and lowered HbA_{1c} in patients with high baseline depression scores up to 1 year of follow-up. Steed et al. [40] described the effect of interventions on psychosocial outcomes including depression, anxiety, adjustment, and quality of life and found that depression seemed to be particularly improved following psychological interventions, while quality of life improved more following self-management. Overall, however, there are few studies that describe approaches that significantly improve self-management and quality of life.

3.3.1   Developing Collaborative Working Practices

It is very easy for families to get into a battle with their diabetes team over less than optimal metabolic control and concerns about nonadherent behavior. Parents may ally themselves on the side of the diabetes team leaving the young person feeling attacked and isolated or alternatively may disagree with the diabetes team and end up with the professional system describing the young person as nonadherent and difficult while the family believes the diabetes team is failing to manage their "difficult diabetes." Young people may be referred to a psychiatrist or other mental health professional which often goes badly, creating frustration and distress and very little change. Families can often feel undermined and ground down by the diabetes. The young person has been living with the diabetes and its effects on their life for many years and parents are often distressed because no intervention seems to have made a difference. Many parents report feeling blamed and criticized for their inability to help their child, and young people often complain that they are held responsible for their illness or for not getting better. The overwhelming and unremitting nature of the distress of some young people can be difficult to remain hopeful about, and we have encountered situations where the problem interferes with the family's and professionals' inclination to collaborate toward the young person's interest.

3.3.2   Establishing Partnerships with Parents and Young People

Children and young people rarely want to see a psychologist and often do not want to talk about diabetes. Paradoxically young people who are struggling with diabetes who may be at the greatest medical risk are often the most difficult to engage [41]. Parents, children, and medical teams may all have different ideas about what they want to get from conversations about diabetes. Inviting people to say what they would like to be different by the end of a consultation enables people to shift their perspective from not knowing what they need to do in order to change but to imagine that things are sorted and to describe what this would look like.

> "As you have come all the way here to meet us today I want to be as helpful as I can be. If this was going to be a helpful meeting, what would be different by the end of our conversation?"
>
> "How do you want to use our time together for it to be helpful?"

For young people who say "don't know" in response to this question, a way of inviting them to join in would be to describe what other people think the problem is and what they might hope for from the meeting. Young people are usually pretty good at telling us what their parents or medical teams want. Parents want children to sort out their "attitude," be aware of potential late effects, or take responsibility for their own care. The medical team wants them to cope better with their diabetes regimen, do more injections or finger pricks, try to not miss injections, or stop eating the "wrong" food.

> "What would your mum/the doctor notice you doing for them to not want you to be coming here?"

3.3.3   Stepping into the Future

We can also invite the family to step into the future when the problem is solved by describing a "preferred future" – how they would like things to look [42]. What would their parents/ friends/teachers be noticing? We also invite parents to tell us what they think they would notice and ask them what they would notice themselves doing or saying differently.

> Jane: I wouldn't have diabetes
> Clinician: So what else would you notice?
> Jane: I wouldn't be arguing with mum about my BM's...
> Clinician: What would you be doing that would help you notice that you weren't arguing?
> Jane: We'd be having breakfast .....maybe (laughing)
> Clinician: What else?
> Jane: I'd be going out with my friends... for a sleepover...going out shopping
> Clinician: What else would you notice?
> Jane: Mum wouldn't be phoning me all the time
> Clinician: What else?
> Jane: I'd feel more confident

Chapter 4
Adolescence

Lorraine Albon

4.1 Introduction

The period of adolescence spans the gap between childhood and adulthood; however setting a precise age range on adolescence can be challenging. The World Health Organization (WHO) defines adolescence as the years between 10 and 19 years [1], as compared to "emergent adulthood" which spans the years between 10 and 25 years. Several policy documents, however, base the provision of healthcare services to young people on the age range 16–19 years.

There are specific changes which occur through the adolescent period which can seemingly make their behavior "challenging" – indeed many adults struggle to relate to young people, irrespective of the added burden of diabetes. This may be because of the negative stereotypes frequently portrayed by the media and the fact that many adults do not have regular contact with youngsters. Both of these factors can make adolescents appear more confusing and frightening than they perhaps really are.

L. Albon
Medical Assessment Unit and Diabetes/Endocrinology Department,
Queen Alexandra Hospital, Portsmouth Hospitals NHS Trust,
Southwick Hill Rd, Portsmouth, Hampshire PO6 3LY, UK
e-mail: lorraine.albon@porthosp.nhs.uk

K.D. Barnard and C.E. Lloyd (eds.), *Psychology and Diabetes Care*, 69
DOI 10.1007/978-0-85729-573-6_4,

There are many physical and emotional changes which occur during adolescence, as children transform into young adults. Physical changes include pubertal development along with the formation of sexual identity and experience. Hormonal changes are occurring at their greatest rate, with the growth hormone in particular being at its height. Most of this activity occurs during sleeping hours, which tends the young person to be easily fatigued. It is perhaps unsurprising that this fatigue may be mistaken for apathy or laziness, both traits frequently associated with "teenagers."

4.2   Psychological and Behavioral Changes

Psychological changes during adolescence include the development of abstract thought, the growth of self-awareness with a set of social constructs, and ideas that are influenced by peers and society in general as much as, or more than, parents [2].

Behavioral changes may involve a shift toward a strong desire for independence coupled with a similar desire for acceptance. Adolescence may be a time of risk-taking behavior, and fitting in with peers can be of paramount importance. Studies have shown that behaviors which are seen as the norm in peer groups can be highly influential in the initiation of risk-taking behaviors [3]. It is at this time that young people develop concepts of personal gain and risk, and somewhere in the chaos, hopefully acquire adequate coping strategies to deal with unforeseen consequences of behavior choices.

Young people may give varied responses to situations such as illness, sometimes reacting with anger, violent outbursts, or noncommunication [2]. These defensive behaviors may be linked to frustration at their perception of being treated like a child at a time when they are frequently told they must take greater responsibility for their own care.

Adolescence and young adulthood may be as much of a challenge for the parents, especially those whose child has had a chronic illness. Evidence suggests that adolescents with a chronic condition are more likely than their peers to engage in risky behavior rather than less [4]. Risk-taking behavior can be testing enough for those parents whose teenagers do not have a chronic illness, and there may be a tendency toward overprotection potentially resulting in conflict.

The way that healthcare teams interact with adolescents and their families is crucial to ensure optimal diabetes control at a time when the endocrine changes associated with puberty may adversely affect control [5], and youngsters with previously exemplary control may struggle with blood sugar regulation.

The pediatric model of care may be very different from that provided to adults – for example, many units operate an open-door policy for children with diabetes to the acute unit – something which is unusual in adult acute care. There may be a highly visible and contactable team of healthcare professionals, many of whom may have been involved with the child since the time of diagnosis, and the move to a different team of healthcare professionals may be difficult. Many healthcare professionals in transitional services report parental difficulties at this time [6].

Top Tips on Talking with Adolescents[1]
- Be warm, positive, authoritative, and respectful.
- Greet appropriately and give time.
- Sit at the same level and observe body language *including your own*.
- Explain, explain, explain!
- Discuss confidentiality in terms the young person can understand.
- Make clear that any information that puts the child at significant risk will be disclosed.
- Ask open questions, one at a time.
- Use the same words but do not mimic "teenage language."
- Summarize what you think you have heard and check back.
- Reflect how the young person seems.
- Show empathy.

---

[1] With thanks to: Dr. Mary Mitchell, Consultant Adolescent Psychiatrist, Hampshire Partnership Trust.

4.3 The Minefield That Is Sex!

4.3.1 Who Does It? Why? At What Age? What Will They Want to Know? What Should We Tell Them?

Despite popular belief, all adolescents are not sexually active. Large international studies have shown that the numbers of young people who have experienced "sexual debut" or who are sexually active are less than one might predict. In 2002, nearly 34,000 students aged 15, from 24 countries, completed an anonymous questionnaire, developed by the HBSC (Health Behaviour in School-aged Children) international research network. The survey showed that the majority of the students had no experience of sexual intercourse, and among those who were sexually active, the majority (82%) used contraception [7].

The figures for the UK were that nearly 38% of 15-year-olds reported having had sexual intercourse, figures which were backed up by a 2008 survey conducted by YouGov for Channel 4 TV [8], which showed that 40% of all 14- to 17-year-olds are sexually active.

The fact that six out of ten 14- to 17-year-olds have *not* had sexual intercourse is a really important point to emphasize not least because many young people feel pressured to indulge in risky behavior as they perceive their peers are similarly engaged. For sexual activity, this, however, is not necessarily true.

There are many factors which are important in predicting sexual activity in young people. Socioeconomic status widely predicts a cross section of early and/or risky behavior [9]. Adolescents from the lowest socioeconomic groups have the highest rates of both alcohol use and teenage pregnancy, both important indicators of the well-being of a younger population.

Although at there may be a wide variation in the prevalence of early sexual debut in different schools, this effect drops when socioeconomic and other cultural factors are taken into account, i.e., if an individual is deprived but attends a school with an affluent catchment, sexual activity may be discouraged [10].

Peer pressure is also a powerful modulator of behavior – having sexually active friends significantly increases the odds that an adolescent's own sexual debut will take place. Nearly 2,500 adolescents in USA were studied in 1994–1995, then again in 1996. Between the two dates, 18% became sexually active, with the higher the proportion of friends who were sexually active, the greater the influence and increased chance of own sexual debut [11].

As young people grow up, the influence of their parents lessens in comparison to that of their peers. Nonetheless, parenting style and attitudes can contribute to the development of risky behaviors, and these factors should be considered when talking to young people about risk [12].

Young people who spend a significant period of time without parental supervision, often after the end of the school day, are more likely to have the opportunity to engage in risky behaviors. In a large US study, those high school students unsupervised for 30 or more hours a week were more likely to be sexually active compared with those who were unsupervised for 5 h a week or less (80% vs. 68%) [13].

While perhaps not directly transferrable to the UK population not least because this study was conducted in a predominately African American population, common sense dictates that the more freedom an young person has, the greater the opportunity for risky behaviors, and opportunities to explore these issues sensitively should be maximized.

Top Tips on Sexual Risk-Taking
- Not everybody is "doing it."
- Never do "it" unless you really want to.
- Always wear a condom.
- Be aware of the effect of alcohol and drugs – they may enable you to do things you might not otherwise consider.

4.3.2   The Impact of Diabetes on Adolescent Sexual Behavior

Around 10% of young adults have a chronic illness such as diabetes, and issues surrounding body confidence over and above those that are prevalent in society in general may be present. It may be thought that these young people have a later sexual debut than their peers although this seems not to be backed up by the literature [14].

There is, however, little literature specific to young people with diabetes, which existing literature sometimes conflicting. One study in 1997 looked at 155 adolescents with type 1 diabetes. The young people represented a wide age group with a study population between 10 and 20 years old. Twenty-nine percent reported unprotected sex; however, this population also reported lower rates for most other risky behaviors when compared to young people without diabetes [15]. The study also highlighted a common finding in that in both groups, the young people perceived the consequences of the risky behavior to be higher for others than for themselves [15].

Conversely, a large study from Italy reported very different findings. Two hundred and fifteen young people with diabetes with a mean age of 14 ± 2 years and with a mean disease duration of 7 ± 5 years were compared to a control group of 464 healthy high school students. It was found that for sexual intercourse, there were similar rates in both groups for young males, 34.8% vs. 35.5%; however young women with diabetes were less likely to have had sex, 29.4% vs. 41.4% [16].

4.3.3   What Will Young People with Diabetes Want to Know About Sex?

Common concerns for young people with diabetes are those surrounding appropriate contraception choices and the effect intercourse may have on diabetes – especially with regard to hypos. Young people may want to discuss the risks of passing on the diabetes to their own children; there may be other issues around sex which are specific to diabetes and can include matters such as female sexual dysfunction and erectile dysfunction in later life for men. It is important that young people are able to express these concerns in an open, caring, and supportive environment.

4.3.4   Contraception Choice

Discussions around contraception should focus not only on the prevention of pregnancy but also on good sexual health. As such, condoms are the contraceptive of choice in this regard. Barrier methods are easily available and have no side effects. There is, however, often extreme embarrassment in both being able to access condoms and in using them. When to negotiate condom use and "putting it on" can be sensitively discussed in clinic to help young adults gain confidence and avoid ineffective and inconsistent use with the potential for failure.

Alternatively, the oral contraceptive pill is safe and effective and available to young women from the age of 16 years. Some young women may struggle to "summon up the courage" to approach their GP for a prescription for the contraceptive pill, and compliance may be imperfect. Frequently cited problems associated with pill use include mood swings and weight gain [17].

Weight gain or the potential for weight gain can be difficult to accept by a body conscious young woman with diabetes, already constrained by the demands of self-management.

Young women with diabetes are recognized as being at risk of eating disorders over and above the general population with the practice of omitting insulin to facilitate weight loss (so-called diabulimia) not an uncommon practice [18].

Many women struggle to take their pill daily, and nearly 50% miss at least one pill per cycle [19].

Young people's lifestyles may be less structured than those experienced in adulthood, thus adherence to medication and treatment advice may be even more problematic. Depo injections are safe and effective, popular with young women, and provide an opportunity for counseling at the point of injection [20].

4.3.5   What Do Young People with Diabetes Choose for Contraception?

Again, the literature is not particularly strong in this area. In 1999, there were fewer women taking the oral contraceptive pill with diabetes than those without the condition, 25% with diabetes compared to 32% without. A third of the women asked said that diabetes influenced their choice of contraception. Interestingly, the pregnancy rate for women aged 25 and over was lower than in the nondiabetic population, while in those less than 25, it was higher – indicating that women with diabetes are less likely to be taking the pill and more likely to have children at a younger age [21].

A more recent study of 89 young women with type 1 diabetes aged between 13 and 19 revealed that half had had unprotected sex. It also showed that over 40% believed that all forms of contraception were less effective when used by women with diabetes and that 69% of girls would feel comfortable asking a professional for contraception [22].

> **Tips for Contraception**
> - Think about it before you need it.
> - Discuss with your GP or family planning clinic.
> - Talk to your partner about it.
> - Carry a condom with you.

4.3.6   "Passing It On"

Young women, in particular, may have concerns about the risk of passing diabetes on to their children and the impact this will have on their future lives but may not discuss these concerns with their diabetes team (see Table 4.1 below). It is crucial that women are provided with the reassurance and support they need, particularly with type 1 diabetes, to be aware that the risk is perhaps not as high as they anticipate.

TABLE 4.1 Risks of passing it on [23]

Type 1 diabetes	Risk (%)
Background rate	0.15
Mother with type 1 diabetes	3
Mothers diagnosed <8 years	13
Fathers	9
Both parents	30
Sibling risk	10
Type 2 diabetes	**Risk (%)**
One parent	15
Both parents	75

4.3.7 Healthy Pregnancies

4.3.7.1 Type 1 Diabetes

It is important to reassure young women that in most cases there is no reason why women with diabetes should not have healthy children. While there may be complicating factors such as a higher incidence of premature ovarian failure in women with type 1 diabetes and polycystic ovaries in those with type 2, these risks should be explored and personalized for the individual. Those with type 1 diabetes have a relative risk malformation of 8% which is 3 times the background rate, but this rises to 12 times the background rate for those with poor control [23].

4.3.7.2 Type 2 Diabetes

Type 2 diabetes is rising in the younger population throughout the world [26] and is associated with increasing levels of obesity, for example, the WHO estimates that in 2007, 10% of English women aged 16–24 were obese [27].

Young women with type 2 diabetes require preconception counseling which may differ from that given to young women with type 1 diabetes. They may be more likely to be significantly obese, have concomitant polycystic ovarian syndrome [28], and may be more likely to have been prescribed teratogenic drugs as they have a higher prevalence of complications such as hypertension and nephropathy than their type 1 counterparts [29].

Counseling should include discussions about contraception, weight management, optimizing blood sugar control and avoidance of potentially harmful medications, statins, and ACE inhibitors as they are more likely to have hypertension.

4.3.7.3   Teratogenic Drugs

Healthcare professionals need to be aware that some drugs commonly used in diabetes are contraindicated in pregnancy and should be stopped or others substituted as soon as family planning occurs [30]. ACE inhibitors may affect fetal and neonatal blood pressure and renal function and can cause skull defects and oligohydramnios. The advice is that these medications should be avoided [30].

Statins affect cholesterol synthesis, and it is this which possibly affects fetal development. There have been reports of limb and midline defects, and again the advice is to avoid these drugs in those seeking conception or to ensure that adequate contraception is in place [31].

There is evidence that many women of childbearing age are prescribed these medications, and their use in the adolescent population is rising, especially with the increasing incidence of type 2 diabetes. In the USA, the provision of beta-blockers and ACE inhibitors has risen from 3.4 per 1,000 in 2004 to 3.8 per 1,000 [32].

NICE clinical guidance 63 diabetes in pregnancy advises that [24]

Starting from adolescence health care professionals should give advice on the benefits of preconception glycaemic control at each contact, that the team should record the woman's intentions regarding pregnancy and contraception use at each contact and that the importance of avoiding an unplanned pregnancy should be an essential component of diabetes education. Those working with young people with diabetes need to feel comfortable discussing preconception care, and there is some evidence that a significant proportion of diabetes nurse educators do not discuss this issue with adolescent women [25].

Key messages from healthcare professionals to women with either type 1 or type 2 diabetes should be given that a healthy pregnancy is a planned pregnancy and that young women contemplating starting a family need to seek preconception counseling to ensure good glycemic control and commence folic acid.

Top Tips for Healthy Pregnancy
- Plan your pregnancy.
- Seek preconception care from your diabetes service.
- Check the drugs you are on are safe in pregnancy.
- If you do get pregnant unexpectedly, seek advice from your GP and diabetes team as soon as you can.

4.3.8   Body Issues

Body confidence in young people with diabetes may be a significant issue – there is increasing evidence that eating disorders are prevalent in young women with type 1 diabetes. This may be related to the constant focus on food, carbohydrate counting, along with the focus on injection sites, etc. This may affect self-image and self-esteem. A third of women say having diabetes has led to loss of self-image. Those with type 1 seem to be more at risk of body issues; 40% of women with type 1 diabetes admit to loneliness and isolation compared to 21% of women with type 2 diabetes; 34% of those with type 1 diabetes state they feel a loss of attractiveness compared to 19% with type 2 [33].

4.3.9   Sexual Dysfunction

Although erectile dysfunction in older men with diabetes is well recognized, female sexual dysfunction is a relatively new phenomenon and can affect younger women. Specific and significant issues are loss of lubrication, loss of sensation, and orgasm difficulty [33].

Young women may have significant issues with sex and may find them hard to talk about. It is important to reassure women that they are not abnormal, that simple measures such as commercially available lubricants are available, and that sharing these difficulties with their partners may also decrease anxiety.

4.3.10   Sex and Hypoglycemia

Although anecdotally sexual activity is known to be a risk factor for hypoglycemia, there is little published literature on this topic. Pragmatic advice should be offered to young people – ensure partners can recognize symptoms of hypoglycemia, that it is a good idea to take a snack to bed and to be aware that the effects of sex, as other exercise, may lead to hypoglycemia some hours after the event.

Top Tips on Sexual Dysfunction and Hypoglycemia
- Sexual dysfunction is common and can be treated.
- Sex does not automatically make you "hypo."
- Be prepared with snacks and bg meter just in case!

4.3.11   Questions to Consider During Consultation

- Have they started a sexual relationship? If not, is it likely to happen and if so are they prepared? Consider carrying a condom.

- Think about the relationship between alcohol and sex – be prepared.
- Contraception – do they know where to get it and how to use it reliably?
- Body issues – do they have concerns about their body – lipohypertrophy? injection sites? pump?
- Are young women having any specific problems with sex which may be associated with diabetes such as loss of lubrication, and do they know what to do or where to get help?
- Are they worried about passing on diabetes?
- Are they worried about having healthy children in the future?
- Do they know that sex can cause hypos? Take a snack to bed and ensure partner knows what to look for.
- Are they planning a pregnancy in the near future? Do they know about preconception clinics? Should teratogenic drugs be stopped?
- Do they know where to get further advice?

4.4 Why Do Young People Smoke, Drink, and Take Drugs?

Despite best medical advice to drink in moderation, avoid drugs, and not smoke, the evidence suggests that these risky behaviors are common among adolescents [34]. The pressure on adolescents to conform to perceived social norms can drive risk-taking behaviors such as these, as can life events and personal experiences. There is evidence that although peer pressure becomes increasingly important as adolescent grows up, parental support and parenting style still has a profound influence on the use of alcohol and other drugs [35].

Conversely, a history of violence within the family, abuse, substance misuse, depression, and perceived stressful life events can increase the likelihood that risky behaviors will occur [36].

Young people are as susceptible to media and advertising as adults, if not more so. Although tobacco advertising has all but disappeared from the TV and cinema, alcohol advertisements are commonplace. An interesting study from the USA explored TV and magazine advertising, in-store advertising, promotional goods, etc., and correlated this with drinking behavior in children in the seventh grade (13 years old). The study reported that the higher the exposure to all forms of advertising, the more likely it was that the seventh grader had already drunk alcohol or intended to do so in the near future. Those in the 75th percentile of alcohol marketing exposure had a predicted probability of drinking which was 50% higher than those in the 25th percentile [37].

A large good-quality systematic review of cohort studies involving over 13,000 people ages between 10 and 26 years old highlighted the fact that many studies did not control for confounders such as parental influence and peer behavior, but note that even so, there remains a correlation between alcohol advertising and drinking behavior. This is likely to confirm and compound the perception that alcohol is associated with "having a good time" "getting into the party mood" [38].

4.4.1 Alcohol: The Extent of the Problem

The European Schools Survey Project looks at young people aged 15–16 every 4 years and has done so since 1995; originally 26 countries took part, but for 2011, 46 countries have expressed an interest in participation. Statistics are available for each participating country and show that for the UK, a large majority (88%) of the students had consumed alcohol during the past 12 months, with more than half (57%) having been drunk during the same period. The estimated consumption on the latest drinking day (6.2 cl alc. 100%) is well above the European mean [34].

4.4.2 Binge Drinking: A Particular Concern

Worryingly, the European Schools project shows that UK teenagers are the highest binge drinkers in Europe. Binge drinking (defined as more than five drinks on more than three occasions in the preceding month) occurs more in girls at about 30% than in boys at about 26%. The older the young person, the higher the likelihood that binge drinking will occur.

While problematic enough in itself, of particular concern is the link between binge drinking, poor school performance, and involvement in other risky behaviors. These include unplanned and unprotected sexual contact, being a passenger in a car where the driver is intoxicated, being the victim of date-related violence, the use of illicit drugs, and even suicide attempts. Furthermore, there appears to be a strong relationship between the frequency of binge drinking and the prevalence of other health risk behaviors. In the USA, binge drinking is said to be involved in the three leading causes of death in young people aged 12–20, namely, accidents, murder, and suicide [39].

Long-term consequences are also a concern, with good evidence that childhood and adolescent drinking predicts alcohol use and alcohol-related problems in adult life. Young people who drink heavily are more likely to become adults who drink heavily [40].

4.4.3 Alcohol and Diabetes

Despite the above, it is naïve to think that young people with diabetes differ significantly from their peers. Evidence shows that while young people with diabetes drink less than their peers who do not have diabetes, levels of alcohol consumption remain above recommended safe limits. Self-reported alcohol use in the general population varies from 39% to 50% of individuals, with approximately 26% of adolescents with T1DM reporting ongoing or sustained alcohol use [41]. This is lower than in healthy control participants: in one study the rates of alcohol use were 30.1% compared to 39.2% in those without diabetes ($p<0.01$). However, while individuals with type 1 diabetes drink less than their healthy peers, this still represents a substantial number of people who engage in this behavior. The likelihood and severity of harm associated with alcohol use is higher in people with diabetes than in the general population.

Hypoglycemia is a specific risk associated with alcohol and diabetes. The perception of hypoglycemia can be lowered even with moderate alcohol consumption, making it less likely that the young person can take action [42]. Alcohol also delays the recovery from a hypo by inhibiting hepatic gluco-neogenesis. This is worsened if the young person is malnourished due to depleted glycogen stores. This may be especially relevant in young women who maintain a low body weight.

Top Tips for Alcohol Consumption
- Never drink on an empty stomach – eat crisps!
- Have a starchy snack before bed – chips/kebab on the way home or cereal/toast when you get in.
- Hypos can be confused with being drunk – tell your mates, wear ID, carry some carbs.
- Think ahead – is there a chance you may want to stay over at a friend's? You should take your long-acting insulin with you. Alcohol can lower your inhibitions, you should carry a condom. Just in case.
- Think about what you're drinking – cocktails and alcopops may be very sugary – you may need a bit more short-acting insulin to cover this.
- Is your drinking becoming a problem? Have you got into trouble with the police? Ended up in the Emergency Department? Done things you would not have done sober?
- Do you know where you can get help if you need it to reduce your drinking?

4.4.4   Specific Questions and Advice for Young People for a Night Out Involving Alcohol

- Ask about their experience of alcohol. Do they drink? How much? How often? Where? Do they binge drink? What do their parents think of alcohol? Is it available at home? Is there a possibility of substance abuse within their family?

- Do they understand the risks of binge drinking? Violence, accidents, unplanned sex, sexual violence?
- Do they understand the effect of alcohol on their diabetes?

4.4.5   Tobacco

In the UK the prevalence of tobacco smoking appears to be on the decline, at least among adults. Smoking fell to its lowest recorded level in 2007 – 21% of the population of Great Britain aged over 16 and 66% of smokers said they wanted to give up [43]. The European Schools project shows smoking is less frequent among young people in the UK than in many other ESPAD countries: the proportion who had smoked during the past 30 days at 22% is below average. While these figures are very positive, of concern is that the highest use of tobacco in the UK today is among young women aged 15–16 [34].

Similar factors are associated with smoking prevalence as are associated with alcohol use. An adverse socioeconomic background, depression, abuse, and violence within families increase the likelihood of tobacco use, and parental style, engagement in school, and out of school activities are protective [36].

4.4.6   Smoking and Diabetes

There is little evidence surrounding tobacco use in young people with diabetes, particularly in the UK. Studies from Europe and the USA give some idea of the prevalence of tobacco use and its association with adverse metabolic parameters in patients with diabetes. An Austrian study looking self-reported smoking status found that self-reported smoking was negligible in patients younger than 11 years, increasing to 5% in 11- to 15-year-old patients and 28% in the

15- to 20-year-old age group. Even after adjustment for age, diabetes duration, sex, and insulin therapy, smokers still had higher HbA1c levels compared with nonsmokers (9.1% vs. 8.0%). Diastolic blood pressure was higher, and lipid profiles were unfavorable [44].

A recent US study demonstrated a lower tobacco use among young people but confirmed the link with metabolic risk. Around 17% of those aged 15–19 with both type 1 and type 2 diabetes used tobacco. Interestingly, a higher proportion of people aged 20 or above with type 2 diabetes smoked than those with type 1, 40% compared with 34% [45]. The risk of tobacco use was greatest in the young people living in families with the lowest incomes and was also correlated with other adverse biomarkers such as raised triglycerides and physical inactivity. Perhaps most worrying is the statistic that fewer than half of young people (aged 10–14 years) reported having received any advice to quit or abstain from smoking by their healthcare team [45].

4.4.7   Smoking Prevention and Cessation in Young People with Diabetes

Young people live in a world of information overload, they are bombarded with advice and can literally take it or leave it.

For a young person, the fact that coronary heart disease is eight times more frequent or that mortality rates are two times higher in smokers with diabetes is relatively meaningless.

Advice needs to be short, accessible, and relevant. There is evidence that a targeted short intervention may encourage young people to stop smoking but is ineffective in preventing them from starting [46].

Given that smoking is a particular problem for young women, a more promising approach is appealing to vanity using facial morphing techniques to show young smokers the effects of smoking on their appearance in the relatively near future. Young women aged 18–24 were shown computer-generated images of themselves as they would become if they continued to smoke. This provoked extreme reactions, they were concerned about other people's reactions to them as older smokers with wrinkled skin, and many experienced physical shock reaction including nausea when seeing how they would age if they continued to smoke. Women reported being highly motivated to stop smoking as a result of the intervention, and many reported that they would take active steps to do so having seen what they would look like if they continued to smoke. This was linked with increased perceived personal responsibility for quitting [47].

Top Tips for Smoking Cessation
- Try very hard not to start.
- If you must, try and limit the number you smoke.
- If you want to stop, seek help from your GP or diabetes clinic.
- Tell everyone you are giving up – they will help keep you on track.
- Try and hang out with nonsmoking friends.
- Try and avoid situations where you will be tempted.
- Put the money you save away and use it to buy yourself a special present.

4.4.8   Specific Questions and Advice for Young People with Diabetes Who Smoke

- Have they ever tried smoking?
- If not do they think they might in the future?
- What are their parent's attitudes to smoking?
- Have they thought about how they might say no without losing face in front of their friends?
- If they smoke, do they do so daily and if so how many? Do they smoke one immediately on waking? (indicates a high level of physiological nicotine addiction)

- Have they thought about quitting?
- Do they know where to get help if they want to stop?
- Have they thought about what they will look like if they carry on smoking? Have they seen any of the computer-generated morphing images?

4.4.9   Other Drugs: Illegal and Legal Highs

ESPAD survey (2007)[34] shows that almost one third (29%) of the British students aged 15–16 had used canna-bis, which is above the ESPAD average, but the use of drugs other than cannabis is infrequent (9%). The rates of use of inhalants (9%) and use of pills in combination with alcohol (7%) are both about average, while the nonpre-scription use of tranquillizers or sedatives is very rare (2%) [34].

4.4.10   Drug Use in Young People with Diabetes

There are only four studies looking at the prevalence of drug use in young people with diabetes and were systematically reviewed [48].

The studies rely heavily on structured questionnaires, and the reported prevalence rates differ from 9% to 29% with a population range between 11 and 25. Cannabis was most popular ranging from about 10% to 28% depending on the study. Under reporting of drug use by young people in clinic is likely to be due to the fear of censure and also perhaps due to the reticence of the healthcare professional who may be uncomfortable discussing such issues.

The use of drugs in patients with diabetes is potentially serious and can indicate an increased risk of death from diabetes and nondiabetes-related events. The Yorkshire Register of Diabetes in Children and Young Adults study looked at over 4,000 cases from 1978 to 2004; 108 deaths were identified – mostly male, with 22% of these arising from accidents or violence, but 16% were from drug misuse, excluding alcohol or insulin [49]. A past history of drug abuse also increases the likelihood of death from an acute event related to diabetes by an odds ratio of 5.7 [50].

Top Tips for Drug Advice
- Drugs are best avoided, but if you want to use them, do not use them on your own.
- Remember the munchies with cannabis; you may need more insulin to cover this.
- Remember the risks of DKA with ecstasy; make sure you drink plenty of fluid (preferably nonalcoholic and nonsugary) and eat regularly.
- Do not ever share a needle with someone, even someone you think you know well.
- Make sure that you have some sort of identification to say you have diabetes, so if you are unwell you can be treated quickly.
- If your drug taking is a problem – get some help – talk to your diabetes nurse, GP, or health advisor.

4.4.11   Specific Drug-Related Issues with Type 1 Diabetes

4.4.11.1   DKA and Control of Diabetes

Drug use may be a precipitant in admission for diabetic ketoacidosis, although many young people may not initially admit to it. In an Australian study of youngsters presenting with DKA, over 50% admitted to drug use – most commonly cannabis, ecstasy, ketamine, benzodiazepines, and heroin in decreasing frequency. Only 20% admitted drug use at presentation but volunteered the information with more targeted and persistent questioning [44].

In the USA, a retrospective study recently demonstrated that cocaine use was the strongest predictor of recurrent DKA [51]. Although studies are few, those with high levels of drug use not surprisingly demonstrate poorer metabolic markers of control, more frequent hospital admissions, and fewer attendances at clinic [52, 53].

4.4.11.2 Ecstasy (Methylenedioxymethylmethamphetamine)

Currently the most popular amphetamine analogue, ecstasy is widely available. Its effect on the serotonergic pathways produces euphoria, but larger doses can have a depressive effect. Hyponatremia which can be profound and fatal may be caused by a combination of polydipsia and syndrome of inappropriate antidiuretic hormone. Ecstasy has an effect on the catecholamine system causing elevation of epinephrine and norepinephrine. These counterregulatory hormones accelerate hyperglycemia by enhancing gluconeogenesis and lipolysis. If there is also relative ketosis due to prolonged dancing without food and the consumption of sugary drinks, DKA can result quickly and be severe [54].

4.4.11.3 Ketamine

Ketamine has become a more common drug of abuse over the last 10 years. It is a calcium channel blocker which acts on excitatory neurotransmitters with dose-dependent effects. Ranging from relaxation to depersonalization, the most significant effects can induce a near-death experience. Occasionally, a state similar to malignant hyperthermia can be precipitated with agitation, tachycardia, raised core temperature, rhabdomyolysis, and seizures – there have been deaths described in the literature as well as metabolic acidosis in the absence of diabetes. Those with diabetes risk a severe DKA with acidosis out of proportion to the ketosis.

4.4.11.4   Cannabis

Cannabis is the most commonly used drug other than tobacco and alcohol in young people. Its availability is widespread, it is relatively cheap, and it had a degree of social, if not legal, acceptance not enjoyed by other drugs. The effects of prolonged and excessive cannabis use and the association with psychosis are well recognized and have led to the drug being reclassified as a class A drug in 2010. There is little direct effect on glucose homeostasis; however, there is evidence that habitual cannabis users have adverse markers of control, partly due to the appetite stimulant effects of cannabis (the munchies) and partly due to a reduced desire to conform to testing and insulin administration.

4.4.12   Legal Highs

There are many substances which are used by young people to attain a high (see Table 4.2 below). Some of these are culturally specific, and their use may be high in certain ethnic groups. Khat is a leaf chewed by Somalis and Yemenis. Its active substance, cathinone, is mildly amphetamine like. Its use in some areas of the UK is increasing. Legal highs and designer drugs have not been studied in relation to specific problems relating to diabetes, either in terms of acute metabolic disturbances or longer-term issues with control.

4.4.13   Where and When? Specific Events May Predict a Higher Chance of Drug Use

Young people may behave quite differently in situations where they are away from home with their peers. Holidays abroad to international nightlife resorts such as Ibiza, Ayia Napa, and Amsterdam may lead to risk-taking behaviors

TABLE 4.2 Legal highs

Stimulants	Deliriants
Caffeine	Datura
Mephedrone (now illegal)	Diphenhydramine
Ephedrine	
Khat	
Hallucinogens/psychoactive	*Depressants*
Salvia divinorum	Alcohol
Hawaiian Baby Woodrose	Diethyl ether
San Pedro cactus	
Ololiúqui	*Inhalants*
Tlitliltzin	Nitrous oxide
Nutmeg	
Ergot	
Toad	
Legal highs and designer drugs	
4.1 Alcohol	
4.2 Kava (Kavalactone)	
4.3 Diethyl Ether	
5 Inhalants	
5.1 Nitrous oxide	
5.2 Nitrites	
6 Opioids	
7 Kratom	

which may be less likely at home. Although not specifically studied in a population of people with diabetes, a survey of over 800 in 2002 revealed that 57% used drugs while away and that binge behavior was more common. The most used drugs were ecstasy, GHB, and cocaine, and those who had returned to these resorts were more likely to use than first timers [55].

The same is true of young people backpacking, in one matched study in the UK and Australia of over 1,000 people, the proportion of people drinking alcohol more than five times a week was around 21% in the UK compared to 40% of those backpacking – drug use at 55% was also higher in Australia than in the UK [56]. It is highly likely that young people with diabetes will want to have the same experiences as their nondiabetic peers, and this may include the use of drugs. It is important that the healthcare professional is seen as nonjudgmental and is able to give advice to minimize harm if and when drug use occurs.

4.4.14   Issues to Discuss with Young People Surrounding Drug Use

- Have they been offered drugs in the past?
- Have they tried drugs and if so do they use drugs regularly?
- Have they thought about how to refuse drugs without losing face with their peers?
- What sort of drugs do they use? How often? How much? Where do they use them, with whom, and how?
- Have they ever got into trouble? With the police? Have they had to attend the emergency department because of drug use?
- Are they planning to go away with friends in the near future?
- Do they know they are more likely to take drugs when they are away than at home?
- Do they have ID if anything should happen to them?
- Do they carry some carbs? A condom?
- Do they know that if they have to use drugs it is best not to do so alone and that needle sharing is obviously a high risk?
- Do they know where to get help with drug use if they need it?

4.4.15 Rock and Roll

Music festivals are increasingly part of the experience of young people, and there is evidence that there are increased opportunities for drug use at festivals compared to the home situation, especially ecstasy, inhalants, and hallucinogens [57].

Top Tips on How to Stay Safe in a Festival [58, 59]
- Download a site map before you go; work out where the important things are – the first aid tent, the toilets, the meeting points, etc.
- Identify your tent – large inflatable helium-filled balloon, wacky colors, etc.
- Take:

  - Identification – MedicAlert or similar jewelry may be crucial in an emergency.
  - Insulin (split it).
  - Cool pack (some can be run under a tap and will stay cool for up to 24 h).
  - Food, more food
  - Money, more money.
  - Solar charger for your phone.
  - Condoms.

- Make contingency plans – if you lose each other, your tent, your money, etc.
- Ask someone to text reminders about your long-acting insulin.
- Think about taking disposable prefilled syringes – your GP can advise.
- Do not inject in the toilets.

Think about you parents, they may be worried – text home at least daily.

4.5   Body Art

"Body art is a term applied to tattooing, scarification and the wearing of jewelry in unusual sites. Body piercing is the perforation of the skin and underlying tissue in order to create a small tunnel in the flesh in which jewelry of one kind or another is placed. Sites pierced include ears, nose, face, tongue, belly button, and genitalia" [60].

The adornment of the body in this fashion is an ancient and cross-cultural practice, and one which is not uncommon in young people today. Body art can carry health-related risks, these can be relatively minor or can lead to significant and disfiguring complications. One study of school-age adolescents identified a prevalence of 20% for piercings and 6% for tattoos although prevalence did vary between regions. Worryingly, 56% of those with body art were underage at the time of application [61]. Unsurprisingly, piercings were most common in girls, but tattoos seemed to be more prevalent in boys, especially those with body issues and younger fathers. In general, boys were less aware of the risks associated with body art and were less likely to seek help when it went wrong.

A large US study looked at body piercings and attitudes among over 200 adolescents aged 16.1 ± 2.8 years. In this population, over 40% had a piercing and perceived the majority of sites acceptable, apart from nipple and genitalia which were deemed acceptable by less than 10% [62].

The young people regarded the practice as minimally risky, and those who had pierced themselves perceived less risk from piercing from a nonprofessional (50%) than those who had their piercings done by a professional (77%).

Body piercings carry particular risks depending on the particular site pierced. The lip and tongue are particular areas prone to problems. A study of 50 patients identified problems from the relatively mild such as hematoma to the severe including sepsis [63], but larger studies have identified long-term damage to the oral mucosa and tooth enamel, depending on the metal used in the stud [64].

Once again, there is little in the literature specific to diabetes – anecdotally, there have been at least two cases of DKA precipitated by tongue piercings (Charlton, personal communication), one of ulceration of the ears after ear piercing [65], and this author has seen one case of severe necrotizing infection at the umbilicus requiring skin grafting. There are currently no case reports of problems associated with tattoos in those with diabetes.

Awareness of issues relating to the piercing of those with diabetes is not high in those professionals performing them. Although many ask about diabetes, the particular issue of hypoglycemia after tongue/lip piercing (due to reduced oral intake) is poor in one study, with few respondents being aware of the different requirements of those with type 1 compared to type 2 diabetes.

Those working with young people who have diabetes need to be aware of the specific risks involved and be able to counsel appropriately – again, it is important to emphasize harm and risk reduction rather than expect a young person to desist from a culturally acceptable method of self-adornment.

Top Tips for Those Undergoing Piercings [66]
- Try and ensure your sugars are as well controlled as possible before you have a piercing.
- High sugars put you at risk of infection.
- Infection can cause your sugars to rise.
- After the piercings, check your sugars at least once a day.
- If your sugars start to rise and you have a fever, pain, or redness at the site or a greeny/yellow discharge, see your doctor as soon as possible; you may need antibiotics.

Mouth and tongue
- Be aware that you may not want to eat afterward as the piercing may be sore.
- You will be at risk of hypos but you should still take your insulin.
- Drink sugary or milky drinks or fruit juice instead.
- Remember to wash your mouth out with water to minimize infection risk.
- If you stop your insulin, your sugars may still go high even if you are not able to eat.

Genital piercings
- Try and make sure your diabetes control is really good beforehand.
- If your sugars are high, you will pass sugar out in the urine, and this may lead to infections.
- This may make your piercing sore and take longer to heal.

References

1. http://www.who.int/topics/adolescent_health/en/index.html.
2. Royal College of Nursing. Adolescence: boundaries and connections – an RCN guide for working with young people. London: RCN; 2008.
3. Kinsman SB, Romer D, Furstenberg FF, Schwarz DF. Early sexual initiation: the role of peer norms. Pediatrics. 1998;102(5):1185–92.
4. Suris JC, Michaud PA, Akre C, Sawyer SM. Health risk behaviors in adolescents with chronic conditions. Pediatrics. 2008;122(5): e1113–8.
5. Dunger DB. Diabetes in puberty. Arch Dis Child. 1992;67(5): 569–70.
6. Shaw KL, Southwood TR, McDonagh JE. User perspectives of transitional care for adolescents with juvenile idiopathic arthritis. Rheumatology (Oxford). 2004;43(6):770–8.
7. Godeau E, Nic Gabhainn S, Vignes C, Ross J, Boyce W, Todd J. Contraceptive use by 15-year-old students at their last sexual intercourse: results from 24 countries. Arch Pediatr Adolesc Med. 2008; 162(1):66–73.
8. Teen Sex Survey. Channel 4. http://sexperienceuk.channel4.com/ teen-sex-survey (2008).
9. Mason WA, Hitch JE, Kosterman R, McCarty CA, Herrenkohl TI, Hawkins JD. Growth in adolescent delinquency and alcohol use in relation to young adult crime, alcohol use disorders, and risky sex: a comparison of youth from low- versus middle-income backgrounds. J Child Psychol Psychiatry. 2010;51(12):1377–85.
10. Henderson M, Butcher I, Wight D, Williamson L, Raab G. What explains between-school differences in rates of sexual experience? BMC Public Health. 2008;8:53.
11. Sieving RE, Eisenberg ME, Pettingell S, Skay C. Friends' influence on adolescents' first sexual intercourse. Perspect Sex Reprod Health. 2006;38(1):13–9.

12. Miller P, Plant M. Parental guidance about drinking: relationship with teenage psychoactive substance use. J Adolesc. 2010;33(1):55–68.

13. Cohen DA, Farley TA, et al. When and where do youths have sex? The potential role of adult supervision. Pediatrics. 2002;110(e6):e66.

14. Suris JC, Resnick MD, Cassuto N, Blum RW. Sexual behavior of adolescents with chronic disease and disability. J Adolesc Health. 1996;19(2):124–31.

15. Frey MA, Guthrie B, et al. Risky behavior and risk in adolescents with IDDM. J Adolesc Health. 1997;20(1):38–45.

16. Scaramuzza AE, De Palma A, Mameli C, Spiri D, Santoro L, Zuccotti GV. Adolescents with type 1 diabetes and risky behaviour. Acta Paediatr. 2010;99(8):1237–41.

17. Robinson SA, Dowell M, Pedulla D, McCauley L. Do the emotional side-effects of hormonal contraceptives come from pharmacologic or psychological mechanisms? Med Hypotheses. 2004;63(2):268–73.

18. Kakleas K, Kandyla B, Karayianni C, Karavanaki K. Psychosocial problems in adolescents with type 1 diabetes mellitus. Diabetes Metab. 2009;35(5):339–50.

19. Rosenberg MJ, Waugh MS, Burnhill MS. Compliance, counseling and satisfaction with oral contraceptives: a prospective evaluation. Fam Plann Perspect. 1998;30(2):89–92, 104.

20. Taflefski T, et al. Contraception in the adolescent patient. Prim Care. 1995;22(1):145–59.

21. Lawrenson RA, Leydon GM, et al. Patterns of contraception in UK women with Type 1 diabetes: a GP data base study. Diabet Med. 1999; 16(5):395–9.

22. Schwarz EB, Sobota M, Charron-Prochownik D. Perceived Access to Contraception Among Adolescents With Diabetes: Barriers to Preventing Pregnancy Complications. The Diabetes Educator. 2010;36(3):489–94.

23. Table Textbook of Diabetes.

24. NICE clinical guideline 63; 2008.

25. Michel B, Charron-Prochownik D. Diabetes nurse educators and preconception counseling. Diabetes Educ. 2006;32(1):108–16.

26. Arslanian S. Type 2 diabetes in children, clinical aspects and risk factors. Horm Res. 2002;57 suppl 1:19–28.

27. http://apps.who.int/bmi/index.jsp.

28. Downs JS, Arslanian S, de Bruin WB, Copeland VC, Doswell W, Herman W, Lain K, Mansfield J, Murray PJ, White N, Charron-Prochownik D. Implications of type 2 diabetes on adolescent reproductive health risk: an expert model. Diabetes Educ. 2010;36(6): 911–9.

29. Eppens MC, Craig ME, Cusumano J, Hing S, Chan AK, Howard NJ, Silink M, Donaghue KC. Prevalence of diabetes complications in adolescents with type 2 compared with type 1 diabetes. Diabetes Care. 2006;29(6):1300–6.

30. Tabacova S, et al. Adverse pregnancy outcomes associated with maternal enalapril antihypertensive treatment. Pharmacoepidemiol Drug Saf. 2003;12(8):633.
31. Edison RJ, et al. Mechanistic and epidemiologic considerations in the evaluation of adverse birth outcomes following gestational exposure to statins. Am J Med Genet A. 2004;131(3):287–98.
32. Liberman JN, et al. Prevalence of antihypertensive, antidiabetic, and dyslipidemic prescription medication use among children and adolescents. Arch Pediatr Adolesc Med. 2009;163(4):389–91.
33. Meeking DR, et al. Assessing the impact of diabetes on female sexuality. Community Nurse. 1997;3(8):50–2.
34. ESPAD. http://www.espad.org/documents (2007).
35. Plant M, Miller P. Young people and alcohol: An international insight. Alcohol Alcohol. 2001;36:513–15.
36. Simantov E, Schoen C, Klein JD. Health-compromising behaviors: why do adolescents some or drink?:identifying underlying risk and protective factors. Arch Pediatr Adolesc Med. 2000;154(10):1025–33.
37. Collins RL, et al. Early adolescent exposure to alcohol advertising and its relationship to underage drinking. J Adolesc Health. 2007;40(6):527–34.
38. Smith LA, Foxcroft DR. The effect of alcohol advertising, marketing and portrayal on drinking behaviour in young people: systematic review of prospective cohort studies. BMC Public Health. 2009; 9:51.
39. Miller JW, et al. Binge drinking and associated health risk behavior among high school students. Pediatrics. 2007;119(1):76–85.
40. McCambridge J, McAlaney J, Rowe R. Adult consequences of late adolescent alcohol consumption: a systematic review of cohort studies. PLoS Med. 2011;8(2):e1000413.
41. Glasgow AM, Tynan D, Schwartz R, Hicks JM, Turek J, Driscol C, O'Donnell RM, Getson PR. Alcohol and drug use in teenagers with diabetes mellitus. J Adolesc Health. 1991;12(1):11–4.
42. Kerr D, et al. Alcohol causes hypoglycaemic unawareness in healthy volunteers and patients with type 1 (insulin-dependent) diabetes. Diabetologia. 1990;33:216–21.
43. Office for national statistics.
44. Hofer SE, Rosenbauer J, Grulich-Henn J, Naeke A, Fröhlich-Reiterer E, Holl RW. DPV-Wiss. Study Group. J Pediatr. 2009; 154(1):20.e1–3.e1.
45. Reynolds K, Liese AD, Anderson AM, Dabelea D, Standiford D, Daniels SR, Waitzfelder B, Case D, Loots B, Imperatore G, Lawrence JM. Prevalence of tobacco use and association between cardiometabolic risk factors and cigarette smoking in youth with type 1 or type 2 diabetes mellitus. J Pediatr. 2011;158(4):594.e1–601.e1.
46. Hollis JF, et al. Teen reach: outcomes from a randomized, controlled trial of a tobacco reduction program for teens seen in primary medical care. Pediatrics. 2005;115(4):981–9.

47. Grogan S, Flett K, Clark-Carter D, Gough B, Davey R, Richardson D, Rajaratnam G. Women smokers' experiences of an age-appearance anti-smoking intervention: a qualitative study. Br J Health Psychol. 2010;16(4):675–89.

48. Lee P, Greenfield JR, et al. Managing young people with Type 1 diabetes in a 'rave' new world: metabolic complications of substance abuse in Type 1 diabetes. Diabet Med. 2009;26:328–33.

49. McKinney PA, Feltbower RG, Stephenson CR, Reynolds C; Yorkshire Paediatric Diabetes Special Interest Group. Diabet Med. 2008;25(11):1276–82.

50. Laing SP, Jones ME, et al. Psychosocial and socioeconomic risk factors for premature death in young people with type 1 diabetes. Diabetes Care. 2005;28:1618–23.

51. Nyenwe EA, Loganathan RS, Blum S, Ezuteh DO, Erani DM, Wan JY, Palace MR, Kitabchi AE. Active use of cocaine: an independent risk factor for recurrent diabetic ketoacidosis in a city hospital. Endocr Pract. 2007;13(1):22–9.

52. Saunders SA, Democratis J, Martin J, Macfarlane IA. Intravenous drug abuse and Type 1 diabetes: financial and healthcare implications. Diabet Med. 2004;21(12):1269–73.

53. Karam GA, et al. Effects of opium addiction on some serum factors in addicts with non-insulin-dependent diabetes mellitus. Addict Biol. 2004;9(1):53–8.

54. Seymour H, et al. Severe ketoacidosis complicated by 'ecstasy' ingestion and prolonged exercise. Diabet Med. 1996;13(10):908–9.

55. Bellis MA, et al. The role of an international nightlife resort in the proliferation of recreational drugs. Addiction. 2003;98(12):1713–21.

56. Bellis MA, et al. Effects of backpacking holidays in Australia on alcohol, tobacco and drug use of UK residents. BMC Public Health. 2007;7:1.

57. Lim MS, et al. Surveillance of drug use among young people attending a music festival in Australia, 2005-2008. Drug Alcohol Rev. 2010; 29(2):150–6.

58. Charlton J, Mackay L. Type 1, tents, take-aways and toilets – how to manage type 1 diabetes at music festivals. Pract Diabetes Int. 2010; 27(7):272–5.

59. http://www.diabetes.org.uk/MyLife-YoungAdults/Living-my-life/Festivals.

60. Denton D, editor. Body Art, cosmetic therapies and other special treatments. London: Chartered institute of environmental health; 2001.

61. Celogon L, et al. The prevalence of body art body piercing and tattoo: awareness of health related risks among 4,277 Italian secondary school adolescents. BMC Public Health. 2010;10.

62. Gold MA, Schorzman CM, Murray PJ, Downs J, Tolentino G. Body piercing practices and attitudes among urban adolescents. J Adolesc Health. 2005;36(4):352.e17–24.
63. De Moor RJ. Dental and oral complications of lip and tongue piercings. Br Dent J. 2005;199(8):506–9.
64. Hickey BM, Schoch EA, Bigeard L, Musset AM. Complications following oral piercing. A study among 201 young adults in Strasbourg, France. Community Dent Health. 2010;27(1):35–40.
65. Antoszewski B, Jedrzejczak M, Kruk-Jeromin J. Complications after body piercing in patient suffering from type 1 diabetes mellitus. Int J Dermatol. 2007;46(12):1250–2.
66. Charlton J, Adamson K, Strachan M, McKnight J. Body piercing: a dangerous practice in Type 1 diabetes. Pract Diabetes Int. 2006; 23(4):166–8.

Chapter 5
Diabetes and Special Groups

Cathy E. Lloyd and Alan Sinclair

Key Points
- Identification of psychological problems in minority ethnic groups living with diabetes can be challenging. It is important for practitioners to have an understanding and awareness of cultural differences in reporting of psychological and emotional well-being in order to provide optimum patient-centered care.
- Current recommendations for the care of women with diabetes before and during pregnancy focus on medical considerations, especially achieving tight blood glucose control in order to reduce the risk of complications during pregnancy and childbirth. However, the psychosocial impact of prenatal care for women with diabetes in pregnancy is less well recognized and has only recently begun to be considered.

C.E. Lloyd (✉)
Faculty of Health & Social Care, The Open University,
Walton Hall, Milton Keynes, MK7 6AA, UK
e-mail: c.e.lloyd@open.ac.uk

A. Sinclair
Institute of Diabetes for Older People,
Beds & Herts Postgraduate Medical School,
Bedfordshire, UK

K.D. Barnard and C.E. Lloyd (eds.), *Psychology and Diabetes Care*,   103
DOI 10.1007/978-0-85729-573-6_5,
© Springer-Verlag London Limited 2012

- The presence of comorbidities in people with diabetes can lead to a substantial increase in the medical management of their condition, and this can also have a significant psychological impact which should not be ignored.
- Diabetes in older adults is a challenging condition that requires insight into the issues of aging, patience in defining the priorities of care, and skills to enhance clinical outcomes.

5.1   Introduction

Individuals can experience diabetes and its comorbidities in a range of ways, and the psychological consequences are varied. Some groups in society have a higher risk of developing diabetes, particularly individuals of South Asian descent, and other groups, for example, older people, may experience greater difficulties with monitoring their diabetes and with the development of diabetes complications. These challenges for 'special groups' of people with diabetes can impact on their psychological well-being and thus have implications for practice. This chapter aims to consider four such 'special groups': older people, women who experience pregnancy and childbirth, individuals from minority ethnic groups, and people with multiple health conditions or 'comorbidities'. Through the consideration of these groups, the chapter highlights the importance of individualized person-centered care which incorporates psychological aspects of diabetes into holistic treatment and care.

5.2   Minority Ethnic Groups

The risk of developing type 2 diabetes is markedly increased in some minority ethnic groups, including South Asians and Afro-Caribbeans [1]. Not only is the prevalence of diabetes much higher in these groups, onset can be earlier and risk of complications much greater [1]. Providing health care to individuals from minority ethnic groups can be challenging, not least because of the cultural and communication difficulties often faced. In particular, healthcare professionals may find it difficult to identify those in need of psychological and emotional support, sometimes because there are communication difficulties, but also because of the stigma attached to mental illness in many communities.

Although there has been a heightened interest in the psychological well-being of people with diabetes in recent years [2, 3], little is known about the existence of psychological problems in minority ethnic groups living with diabetes in the UK [4]. Feeling depressed can impact on the ability to self-care and lead to poor glycemic control, increased risk of diabetes complications, and poor quality of life [5]. Clinically diagnosed major depressive disorder is only one end of the spectrum of depression, with lower symptom levels being more common although still having a debilitating effect on the individual. In one of the few published studies conducted in the developing world, nearly a fivefold increase in the prevalence of clinically significant levels of depression in men and a doubling of rates in women with diabetes (compared to those without diabetes) have been reported [6]. A trebling of prevalence rates has been observed in people with diabetes in Pakistan compared to people without diabetes [7].

Recent guidelines have stressed there is an underestimation of psychological distress in South Asians, compounded by negative perceptions and stigma surrounding mental illness in this diverse group, along with a lack of awareness of available support [8]. A Department of Health report on mental health care cites cultural differences in beliefs and practices, language barriers, and broader social risk factors as all important in addressing inequalities in mental healthcare service use [9].

A number of established screening tools for depression have been translated into different languages or have been used in different countries. Although these may be useful in some settings, it is important to note that there have been concerns noted with regard to the cultural applicability of these tools and the appropriateness of direct language translations [10]. Direct translations of screening tools from one language (usually English) to another may be problematic. Usually, the screening tool in question is translated and back-translated by different people, and this is followed by a discussion around any discrepancies so that a consensus may be reached as to the final content. Notwithstanding the importance of clarity in the actual procedure of translation, there may be difficulties in the degree of conceptual proximity between the original questionnaire and the language it is to be translated into.

In order to develop a valid translation the translators must have an in-depth knowledge of both cultures. This is important, particularly as symptoms of mental distress may have a different level of significance or meaning in different cultural groups or may have differing sources or impact. Somatic symptoms may be more commonly reported in some cultures, and this has particular resonance in regard to physical health and any potential overlap with the symptoms of diabetes. On the other hand, cognitive items, for example, fear about the future or feelings of hopelessness, may be confounded not only with external environmental features in peoples' lives but also with concerns about diabetes-related events, such as the development of complications such as loss of sight, heart disease, and so on. It has been argued that for many migrants (especially those who have experienced a degree of acculturation), the use of screening tools from an original culture may be no better or worse than using one from the host culture [10]. However, this may depend on the questionnaire used and the particular concepts or sources of distress contained therein.

In the UK, there are now clear recommendations for the identification of depression in primary care [11]. The National Institute of Health and Clinical Excellence (NICE) states that 'diabetes professionals should ensure they have appropriate skills in the detection and basic management of non-severe psychological disorders in people from different cultural backgrounds...' [11]. The Quality and Outcomes Framework recommends the use of two screening questions (see the box below), followed by a brief questionnaire if required, to identify people with depressive symptoms in need of treatment.

> Quality and Outcomes Framework recommended two screening questions for use in general practice:
> 1. During the past month have you often been bothered by feeling down, depressed or hopeless?
> 2. During the past month have you often been bothered by little interest or pleasure in doing things?
> Arroll et al. [12], Whooley et al. [13]

The most commonly used instrument to measure level of depression in primary care is the Patient Health Questionnaire (PHQ-9), developed in the USA [14]. However, although this instrument is appropriate for English-speaking (and writing) individuals, its utility in groups where literacy might be a problem and also its cultural applicability are unclear. Indeed, although a small amount of work has been done translating written self-report instruments designed to measure depression, to date, there has been a lack of research into validating these, especially for South Asians with diabetes living in the UK [4]. In our research, we have recently begun to address the cultural applicability of the PHQ-9 in South Asians with diabetes, many of whom are not literate and speak a language that does not have an agreed written form, for example, Sylheti (spoken in Bangladesh) and Mirpuri (spoken in particular regions of Pakistan). We asked focus group participants to describe how they felt and what the concept of depression meant to them; some of their responses are shown in the box below.

What does depression mean to you?
'I think it is some sort of pain deep in your heart or pain in the head you can feel pain but it is difficult to explain to others'
'It happens sometimes to me... a feeling of tiredness and pain'
'More or less a feeling of helplessness .... It affects my daily activities'
'Well I actually feel some kind of heaviness in my heart, when I am upset'

Some research has suggested that there may be a particular 'language of emotions' in certain ethnic groups, which might be more related to the somatic symptoms of depression or psychological distress [15]. Our research supports this, as the quotes above demonstrate. The use of idioms in questionnaires is especially problematic, for example, 'feeling blue,' 'feeling low,' and 'butterflies in the stomach' may lose their meaning, and attempts to find conceptually equivalent items or expressions which describe mental distress may be difficult. Some of the scales used to measure the frequency or intensity of symptoms may also be difficult to translate. Indeed, some research has indicated that rather than using options such as 'rarely,' 'sometimes,' 'frequently,' etc., a color-coded visual analogue scale may be more appropriate [16]. An example of a scale we have developed for use with the PHQ-9 is shown below (Fig. 5.1).

A 'positive' rather than a 'negative' scale for screening for psychological well-being may be more appropriate or more acceptable to some individuals. A good example of this is the WHO-5 well-being scale which has been shown to be reliable in identifying individuals with symptoms of depression [17, 18]. Recently, we have developed a color-coded scale for use with the WHO-5 and have found high acceptability in individuals with diabetes from South Asian backgrounds (Fig. 5.2).

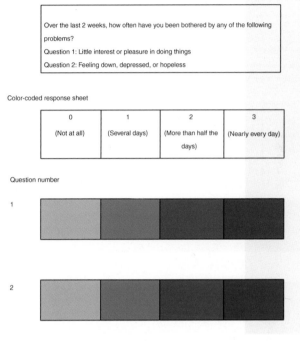

Over the last 2 weeks, how often have you been bothered by any of the following problems?

Question 1: Little interest or pleasure in doing things

Question 2: Feeling down, depressed, or hopeless

Color-coded response sheet

0	1	2	3
(Not at all)	(Several days)	(More than half the days)	(Nearly every day)

Question number

1

2

FIGURE 5.1 Example questions from the PHQ-9 using a color-coded visual analogue scale

Self-complete instruments are not always appropriate in populations where there is a high prevalence of illiteracy or where the main language does not have an agreed written form and is only spoken [19]. Visual analogue scales, used in conjunction with an audio version of the screening tool or an oral administration of the questionnaire, can go some way to address these difficulties.

Other aspects of psychological distress are also important, for example, anxiety about different treatment regimens, testing blood sugar levels, or fear of hypoglycemia. For some people from minority ethnic groups, these worries and concerns may be compounded by language barriers and misunderstandings between healthcare professionals and individual

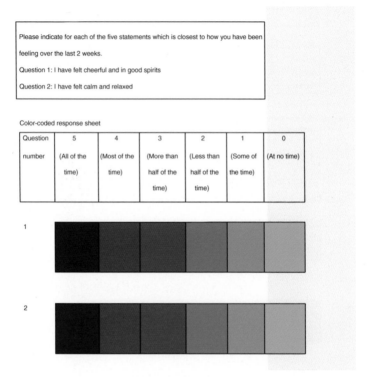

Please indicate for each of the five statements which is closest to how you have been feeling over the last 2 weeks.

Question 1: I have felt cheerful and in good spirits

Question 2: I have felt calm and relaxed

Color-coded response sheet

Question number	5 (All of the time)	4 (Most of the time)	3 (More than half of the time)	2 (Less than half of the time)	1 (Some of the time)	0 (At no time)
1						
2						

FIGURE 5.2 WHO-5 – Example questions and color-coded response sheet

patients. Translators are not always available in diabetes clinics, and cultural beliefs may make it difficult to discuss problems with self-care or other aspects of their personal life with the diabetes team. Research has suggested that there may be benefits for both the individual patient and members of the healthcare team if the latter understood more about the positive aspects of culture and any impact on diabetes care [20].

Although cultural and communication difficulties often make appropriate support of self-management of diabetes more difficult, these are not insurmountable [19,21]. Research has demonstrated that the use of Asian support workers, or Asian link workers, markedly improves patient outcomes in terms of increased knowledge and understanding of their diabetes and improved attendance rates at clinics and at education sessions [22]. An understanding of cultural difference is important. However, it is vital that difference is not assumed on the basis of appearance or language. Diversity is present within as well as between different cultural groups, and an understanding of individual needs and concerns remains key if self-care is to be optimized.

Tips for Practice
- Each patient will report their emotional well-being in a different way – culture, age, language, and gender are some of the factors that should be considered.
- Some individuals will be comfortable with answering the two standard screening questions, others will not. Similarly, the use of the PHQ-9 (or other questionnaires) will be acceptable to some patients and not others.
- It is important to address the individual needs of each patient – for example not all patients from a South Asian background have the same needs for psychological care.

5.3 Pregnancy and Diabetes

During pregnancy and childbirth, diabetes introduces a range of challenges for both the women themselves and those providing their care. Current recommendations for the care of women with diabetes before and during pregnancy focus on medical considerations, especially achieving tight blood glucose control [23]. The main aim of this care is to reduce the risk of complications during pregnancy and childbirth. However, the psychosocial impact of prenatal care for women with diabetes in pregnancy is less well recognized and has only recently begun to be considered. In this section of the chapter, we consider both the medical and the psychosocial challenges related to experiencing and providing care for women with diabetes during pregnancy.

Diabetes is the most common medical complication in pregnancy and is associated with an increased risk of obstetric complications, including congenital abnormalities, increased rates of caesarean delivery, and perinatal mortality [24]. Rates of diabetes during pregnancy are rapidly increasing and are seen to be a serious public health concern [24]. These increased rates are mainly due to the rapid rise in the numbers of women who have type 2 diabetes, and it has been suggested that this is associated with an increased prevalence of overweight and obesity [25]. Gestational diabetes (GDM) – onset of diabetes during pregnancy – occurs when the body cannot produce enough insulin to meet the extra needs of pregnancy. It is associated with being overweight and also with a family history of type 2 diabetes. Although it usually goes away after childbirth, women with GDM have an increased risk of developing type 2 diabetes later on in life as well as having GDM in subsequent pregnancies. Both type 2 diabetes and GDM are more common in women from minority ethnic groups, and there may be differences in the experiences of pregnancy according to ethnicity [26]. For example, Katbamna [27], who focused on the distinctive cultural practices of Gujarati and Bangladeshi women having babies in the UK, argued that services did not always recognize women's distinct cultural preferences. Other research has indicated that there are cultural differences in experience, with South Asian women being more influenced by family and religion compared to their white Caucasian counterparts [28, 29].

A key report from the Confidential Enquiry into Maternal and Child Health (CEMACH), which focused on women with preexisting diabetes, highlighted a fivefold increase in stillbirths, a threefold increased risk of perinatal mortality, and a twofold increased risk of congenital abnormalities [30]. Preterm delivery rates were more than five times more common in women with diabetes compared to women without this condition, and caesarean section rates were nearly trebled. Research suggests that women who develop gestational diabetes also have an increased risk of morbidity and mortality [31], including hypertension, and adverse neonatal outcomes including prematurity, low Apgar scores, and perinatal mortality. However, adverse outcomes are more significant for women with preexisting diabetes compared to women who develop diabetes in pregnancy. The concerns noted in the CEMACH report are reflected in the current NICE recommendations that screening for gestational diabetes should be offered to women with certain identified risk factors, including a body mass index over 30 and any first degree relative with diabetes [23].

While clinical outcomes for both mother and child remain poorer for women with diabetes compared to those without diabetes, there are some signs that diabetes management during pregnancy is improving [32]. Two years ago, NICE issued guidance for the care of women with diabetes during pregnancy which included the physiological and biomedical management of diabetes before, during, and after pregnancy. There is evidence to suggest that such management reduces both neonatal and maternal morbidity and mortality [33, 34]. These guidelines have paved the way to more standardized care by providing a template for care protocols throughout the UK. However, recent research suggests that although diabetes management in pregnancy might be improving, this improvement is not uniform across the UK [35].

The psychosocial impact of having diabetes during pregnancy is less well researched and may often be ignored. Having diabetes means having to incorporate a whole range of self-care behaviors into daily life including blood testing, medication taking, and following a healthy diet. These self-care behaviors are coupled with the increased surveillance of women with diabetes during pregnancy, recommended in order to improve outcomes for both mother and child. These factors alter the experience of mothers-to-be, placing them into a category of 'at risk' and experiencing a medicalized pregnancy and birth. This can reinforce feelings of being 'different' from other pregnant women, especially when mothers do not have access to a community midwife but are only seen in secondary care. Our experiences with mothers-to-be have suggested that use of a 'buddying' system can be helpful and reduce feelings of isolation as well as demonstrating that successful outcomes are achievable.

Although remaining almost exclusively focused on biomedical care, the NICE guidance on diabetes in pregnancy acknowledges the need to 'take into account women's needs and preferences.' The report suggests that 'Women with diabetes should have the opportunity to make their informed decisions about their care and treatment, in partnership with their healthcare professionals' (NICE [23], p. 6).

This is not to say that women want their biomedical and physiological needs ignored or even placed as secondary. Indeed, women have considerably high expectations of maternity care services in relation to its ability to reduce, or eradicate, fetal abnormalities or neonatal mortality and morbidity [36], especially following prior experiences of pregnancy loss [37]. Rather, many women report their concern to *integrate* the two aspects so that a more holistic approach to care is promoted.

There are several key areas where the psychological impact of having diabetes during pregnancy need to be considered, including:

- Diagnosis of gestational diabetes
- Preconception care for women with diabetes prior to pregnancy
- Postnatal follow-up and risk of future diabetes
- Self-care during and after pregnancy – an empowerment approach to care

Diagnosis of gestational diabetes can have a significant impact with increased anxiety levels as mothers-to-be cope with this information and learn how to self-manage their condition. As noted above, diabetes imposes a range of care needs on the person with the condition. In pregnant women, this means having to incorporate self-management behaviors such as frequent blood testing and medication taking into their daily lives, which have hitherto not been part of their experience. At the same time, they can expect to be closely monitored by a range of healthcare professionals throughout their pregnancy. Biomedical concern for the well-being of both mother and baby is not without its challenges, however, and women's psychosocial well-being may be compromised. Thus the healthcare team need to be aware of the psychological needs of mothers-to-be.

Not all women with preexisting diabetes plan their pregnancies or indeed attend preconception counseling and/or diabetes education programs prior to becoming pregnant [28]. However, there are data to show that there are great benefits to preconception care, demonstrated by significantly lower congenital malformation rates [28]. Appropriate care for women with preexisting diabetes is not always available, which means the overall risk for poor pregnancy outcomes is even greater. The picture is further complicated by the fact that poorer outcomes are found in women from more socially deprived areas who are less likely to attend preconception clinics [28]. Clearly, there remain serious challenges in encouraging women to attend for preconception care and ensuring its applicability to women from diverse social and ethnic backgrounds.

Women with gestational diabetes are significantly more likely to have this condition in subsequent pregnancies, and they are at increased risk for type 2 diabetes in the future [38]. Examples of good practice include holding postnatal group meetings for mothers 3–6 months after giving birth, where information on diet, exercise, and risk reduction can be disseminated and further support given. However, it may not be appropriate to discuss psychological well-being in any depth during these sessions, given the sensitive nature of this information. Furthermore, not all women attend these sessions, especially those from minority ethnic groups, where language and communication may be difficult. Nevertheless, evidence shows that lifestyle interventions can make a difference [39], although not universally applicable or indeed acceptable to all women.

In the UK, the National Service Framework for diabetes highlighted the importance of optimizing the outcomes of pregnancy through empowering and supporting women with diabetes:

Standard 9: The NHS will develop, implement and monitor policies that seek to empower and support women with pre-existing diabetes and those who develop diabetes during pregnancy to optimise the outcomes of their pregnancy. (Department of Health, 2001 [40])

The principle of empowerment in diabetes care is based upon people taking more control of their care, both for themselves as individuals, and also for others being involved in determining local services and priorities [41]. An empowerment approach to care takes into account social, psychological, and environmental factors are well as medical ones. Anderson and Funnell (2001) have compared two models of diabetes care, which are reproduced in Table 5.1 below.

TABLE 5.1 Two models of diabetes education

The empowerment model	The traditional model
1. Diabetes is a biopsychosocial illness	1. Diabetes is a physical illness
2. Relationship of provider and patient is democratic and based on shared expertise	2. Relationship of provider and patient is authoritarian based on provider expertise
3. Problems and learning needs are usually identified by the patient	3. Problems and learning needs are usually identified by professional
4. Patient is viewed as problem solver and caregiver, i.e., professional acts as a resource and helps the patient set goals and develop a self-management plan	4. Professional is viewed as problem solver and caregiver, i.e., professional responsible for diagnosis and outcome
5. Goal is to enable patients to make informed choices. Behavioral strategies are used to help patients experiment with behavior changes of their choosing. Behavior changes that are not adopted are viewed as learning tools to provide new information that can be used to develop future plans and goals	5. Goal is behavior change. Behavioral strategies are used to increase compliance with recommended treatment. A lack of compliance is viewed as a failure of patient and provider
6. Behavior changes are internally motivated	6. Behavior changes are externally motivated
7. Patient and professional are powerful	7. Patient is powerless, professional is powerful

Anderson and Funnell (2001).

They compared an empowerment model with what they called a 'traditional model' of care and identified the differences in styles of care in terms of providing diabetes education. Diabetes education, usually provided by nurses, is the cornerstone of diabetes care and includes not only knowledge and information dissemination but skills and confidence building in order for each individual to feel able to carry out diabetes self-care activities. These principles are applicable to all individuals with diabetes, not least to women with diabetes during pregnancy.

The use of an empowerment approach to diabetes care may seem straightforward to some practitioners. However, for others, given the huge variability in patient need, type of diabetes care regimen, and external factors that might influence self-care, the implications may seem daunting. It implies that during each consultation between the person with diabetes and a healthcare professional, a dialogue should take place during which these factors can be taken into account, and suggests that all those involved are able to communicate effectively within the time constraints of a consultation. However, the CEMACH report highlighted problems in communication between professionals and women, as well as between different professionals and also deficiencies in standards of note-keeping. In order to address this, the Perinatal Institute (www.pi.nhs.uk) has developed 'Diabetes in Pregnancy Notes' to be used in addition to standard handheld 'Pregnancy Notes' [42]. The idea behind this is to ensure that mothers-to-be are given additional information related to their specific care requirements. These notes also aim to facilitate a partnership approach between the mother and the multidisciplinary team providing care which should help to allay any anxiety and support women in feeling more empowered as regards their care.

In summary, the current recommendations for care for women with diabetes during pregnancy include an increased level of monitoring, both personally and also at the diabetes clinic. These recommendations are aimed at optimizing outcomes for women, both in terms of their baby as well as their risk of developing type 2 diabetes later on in life. However, they may have a negative impact on the personal experience of pregnancy and childbirth. The psychological consequences of having diabetes when pregnant need to be recognized, and appropriate support given at all stages of pregnancy and child-birth. Challenges still remain, however, in terms of putting these recommendations into practice and achieving successful clinical outcomes in pregnancy alongside psychosocial ones.

Tips for Practice
- It is important that both the medical and the psycho-social aspects of care are considered when caring for women with diabetes during pregnancy.
- The use of a 'buddying' system can be helpful and reduce feelings of isolation as well as demonstrating that successful outcomes are achievable.
- A partnership approach to care between the mother and the multidisciplinary team providing care should help to allay any anxiety and support women in feel-ing more empowered as regards their care.

5.4   Comorbidity

Many people with diabetes, especially older people, will experience a degree of complexity of illness that can be very challenging even to the most dedicated health professional. This complexity results from the metabolic condition itself often being exacerbated by a compounding insulin-resistant state, a propensity for vascular complications that can disable (such as peripheral vascular disease or peripheral neuropathy), and the number and severity of associated medical comorbidities.

The term 'comorbidity' has several definitions [43], but in the context of diabetes, it generally refers to a coexisting medical condition that may or may not be caused or associated with the primary condition (in this case, diabetes). The importance of a comorbid illness lies firstly in the experience of the individual person with diabetes whose quality of life may deteriorate. Secondly, the existence of comorbidities means that additional clinical management is required to optimize diabetes care (e.g., use of antihypertensive or lipid-lowering agents), often leading to side effects of this added treatment, a realignment of treatment goals if the comorbidity is severe, and an increase in the experience of disability that may arise from the comorbidity itself. Given these additional requirements for treatment and care as well as the possible effects on quality of life, the potential negative psychological impact on the individual is clear.

Several recent studies have explored varying aspects of diabetes and medical comorbidity. In one study [44], the presence of musculoskeletal disorders, often not included in disease profiling by clinicians, was observed to have a significant impact on activity limitations in those with diabetes. In a US study of older adults (aged > 75 years) [45], the presence of obesity or coronary heart disease was associated with less likelihood of individuals meeting current recommendations on activity levels to maintain health. In another study of people with diabetes and psychiatric disease [46], the presence of alcohol and drug abuse/dependence as comorbidities significantly increased mortality. A study of Australian veterans [47] demonstrated that the presence of various comorbidities such as depression, chronic obstructive pulmonary disease, dementia, or Parkinson's disease, decreased the likelihood of treatment progression for diabetes which in itself may have adverse consequences for individual patients. This may be reflected in suboptimal symptom control, undertreatment of key clinical manifestations, decreased quality of life, and failure to reach an anticipated level of health status.

A number of comorbidity measures are available, but the Charlson Index is often used [48] to provide the clinician with some guidance on the intensity of treatment that might be required. The index provides a 10-year risk prediction of mortality based on the presence of 1 or more of 22 conditions such as heart disease or cancer. These indices, which may have limited utility in individual patients, provide some objectivity of the influence of comorbidities in a patient's healthcare pathway.

The presence of frailty as a comorbidity often has a major impact on health status, treatment decisions, and prognosis. This is a multidimensional syndrome associated with functional decline and increased vulnerability to poor health outcomes [49]. Objective measures usually involve items such as levels of activity, gait speed, hand grip, fatigue, weakness, and weight loss. Diabetes appears to be overrepresented in people with frailty [50], accounting for 25% of participants in the Cardiovascular Health Study [49]. Further work by the same group indicates that insulin resistance may be a precursor to the development of frailty [51].

Several medical comorbidities in people with diabetes can have a significant influence on subsequent progression of disease and prognosis. Apart from renal disease, lipid abnormalities, and hypertension, cardiovascular disease per se is likely to be the most important. Diabetes mellitus has been recognized as an independent major cardiovascular risk factor for more than 30 years. Cardiovascular disease remains the most common cause of death in all age groups of people with diabetes [52]. Diabetes constitutes a mortality risk similar to those of people without diabetes but with previous history of myocardial infarction [53]. Cardiovascular risk factors rarely occur in isolation but rather tend to cluster in what is known as the 'metabolic syndrome'. This is characterized by a group of risk factors including visceral obesity, dyslipidemia {low high density lipoprotein cholesterol (HDL), high triglycerides}, hypertension, impaired glucose/insulin homeostasis (insulin resistance, hyperinsulinemia, glucose intolerance), increased cardiovascular oxidative stress, impaired endothelial function, and abnormal coagulation and fibrinolytic profiles [54]. In the Third National Health and Nutrition Examination Survey [NHANES III], there was an incremental increase in prevalence of the metabolic syndrome with worsening glucose tolerance from 26% in those with normal fasting glucose rising to 86% in those with diabetes [55]. The following case study highlights the complexity of the experience for those with comorbidities and suggests that there may be serious negative psychosocial consequences for some individuals.

Case Study

Mr. Begum was a 71-year-old South Asian gentlemen referred to a hospital diabetes clinic by his GP for management of his poor glycemic control. He had been diagnosed with type 2 diabetes 3 years previously and was taking metformin 850 mg twice daily and indicated that he was following dietary advice given by his GP. His latest HbA1c was 8.9%. He had continued to smoke since his diagnosis of diabetes.

Careful history taking revealed many dietary indiscretions, a lack of blood glucose monitoring, and a reliance on his wife for day to day care. Mr. Begum's blood pressure was raised, his BMI was 32, cholesterol was 5.6 mmol/l, and triglycerides 2.8 mmol/l. His estimated GFR was 62, and he had diminished peripheral leg pulses.

He was considered to have type 2 diabetes, hypertension, lipid dyslipidemia, with evidence of peripheral vascular disease. This was interpreted to also indicate features of the metabolic syndrome. Review by a hospital dietician was arranged; he and his wife received educational support and advice from the community diabetes team, and he was prescribed pioglitazone and an ACE inhibitor. His GP asked to arrange an ankle-brachial measurement to assess his leg circulation, and he was advised to stop smoking.

Eight weeks later, he was self-monitoring and his condition had improved: HbA1c was 7.9%, BMI 29, BP 152/82, with improvements seen in other variables. However, in spite of these improvements in some aspects of his condition, when talking with the dietician, Mr. Begum indicated how overwhelmed he felt with having to take so much new information on board and the impact of having to take all these tablets each day.

After a long discussion, the dietician suggested he could try and take regular exercise by walking 25 min each day if possible as one way of improving his overall level of well-being. However, if his low mood and anxiety did not improve, further input from the diabetes specialist nurse would be available, along with an assessment of his mental health.

It can be appreciated that the presence of a significant comorbidity can have a profound effect on individual case management: in the case of cardiovascular disease and hypertension, this may take the form of altered glucose-lowering therapy (avoiding weight-increasing treatments such as sulphonylureas), which may worsen cardiovascular health status and treatment of associated hypertension, or use of pioglitazone which may have cardiovascular benefits and use of antihypertensives that enhance renal function such as ACE inhibitors. From the individual patient's perspective, these increases in the medical management of their condition can also have significant psychological impact which should not be ignored.

Tips for Practice
- It is important to appreciate the impact of comorbid illness on the experiences of the individual with diabetes whose quality of life may deteriorate.
- The existence of comorbidities means that additional clinical management is often required in order to optimize diabetes care – this may lead to additional side effects.
- A realignment of treatment goals may be necessary if the comorbidity is severe.
- Given these additional requirements for treatment and care as well as the possible effects on quality of life, the potential negative psychological impact on the individual is clear.

5.5   Diabetes and Older People

Within Europe, diabetes affects 10–25% of older adults and results in more frequent clinic visits, higher hospital admission rates, and increased healthcare expenditure [56]. There are a number of implications for care in older people with diabetes including the following key areas of importance:

1. Maintaining a major emphasis on quality of life and well-being for each older person with diabetes
2. Anticipating or planning early and effective interventions
3. Ensuring there is a commitment within your healthcare team to improve and/or *maintain* functional status
4. Avoiding ageism and a reductionist approach to care

5.5.1   What Makes Diabetes in Older Adults a Special Group?

Older people may have concerns in a range of areas around social structures, financial dependency, limited mobility and access to healthcare services, and lowered reserve to illness and infection due to frailty and to the effects of the aging process. In addition, the following may also play a part in altering the healthcare team's approach to care:

- High levels of medical comorbidity (see above)
- Physiological aging and lowered counterregulation to hypoglycemia
- Higher frequency of depressive illness or cognitive impairment
- Nursing home residency
- Greater reliance on informal/formal caregivers
- Increased adverse drug event risk from polypharmacy

These influences are likely to alter a treatment strategy for a patient by one of three ways:

(a) They may guide you and the patient/carer to agreeing a particular achievable/relevant set of care goals.

(b) You are now better placed to prescribe glucose-lowering therapy that emphasizes minimizing vascular complications (where appropriate), avoiding hypoglycemia, and enhancing patient safety.

(c) You should have enough information from examining these influences to plan a structure of care that maintains functional independence, minimizes hospital admission, and supports an empowerment approach to care.

A significant issue that warrants special mention in this section is cognitive dysfunction and diabetes in older people.

5.5.2   Cognitive Dysfunction and Diabetes

Diabetes mellitus and dementia-like illness are common long-term prevalent disorders occurring in the community often enough to coexist in the same individual, although during the last 15 years, there has been increasing evidence from epidemiological and clinical trials that diabetes and cognitive dysfunction are related [57, 58]. The overall risk of dementia appears to be significantly increased for both men and women with type 2 diabetes. In addition, poor glucose control may be associated with cognitive impairment, which recovers following improvement in glycemic control. For example, in a study of people with diabetes aged 70 years and over who were screened for cognitive dysfunction with the Mini Mental State Examination (MMSE) and a clock-drawing test (CDT) [59], it was shown that CDT scores were inversely correlated with HbA1c, suggesting that cognitive dysfunction is associated with poorer glycemic control. A systematic review of prospective studies aiming to evaluate the extent to which diabetes is associated with cognitive decline and dementia [60] has concluded that compared with diabetes-free individuals, people with diabetes have a 1.5-fold greater risk of cognitive decline, a 1.6-fold greater risk of developing dementia, and a greater rate of decline in cognitive function.

The link between diabetes and cognitive dysfunction:
- Professional and public concern about the impact of diabetes on cognition
- Long-term influence about the effects of hyperglycemia and hypoglycemia on cerebral function unknown
- Pathophysiological mechanisms unclear, but may involve vascular, inflammatory, and neuronal mechanisms
- No current agreement on the most optimum method to detect or assess cognitive deficits in diabetes
- Clinical relevance of the changes uncertain

This work (European Diabetes Working Party for Older People (EDWPOP), Clinical guidelines for type 2 diabetes, 2004) can be accessed via the Institute of Diabetes for Older People (IDOP) website: instituteofdiabetes.org.

There is increasing awareness by the profession and the public that diabetes influences memory and the ability to calculate. The background to these developments is summarized in the box above.

The effects of disturbed cognitive function include poorer self-management of diabetes treatment, increasing glucose levels because of inconsistent timing of meals and medication, and increasing risk of hypoglycemia if patients forget that they have taken their hypoglycemic medication and repeat the dose. Cognitive dysfunction in older people with diabetes may remain undetected for some time with symptoms of memory loss, changes in behavior, and disorientation simply being interpreted as 'getting old' or 'eccentricity.' However, a number of considerable implications may result such as increased hospitalization, less ability for self-care, less likelihood of specialist follow-up, and increased risk of institutionalization.

5.5.3 Depression Must Be Excluded in the Evaluation of Cognitive Function in Diabetes

Diabetes mellitus appears to be significantly associated with depression, independent of age, gender, or presence of chronic disease [61], and there is a twofold increased risk of depression when diabetes is present [3, 62]. Cognitive performance scores are likely to be diminished and create difficulties of interpretation for the clinician if a patient has a coexisting depressive state. The relapsing, often unstable nature of depression may exacerbate the difficulty of maintaining good glucose control and taking medications [63]. For frail and housebound individuals, the burden on both formal and informal carers is likely to increase substantially if depression is present. Failure to recognize depression can be serious since it is a long-term, life-threatening, disabling illness and has a significant impact on quality of life [64].

It is important that at the initial assessment patients undergo a thorough history and examination and, in particular, be asked about symptoms of depression and then have one of several mood screening tests, which are now widely available in primary care. If a significant mood disorder is detected, the patient can either be directly treated or referred for specialist assessment [65].

In summary, diabetes and cognitive dysfunction are likely to be interrelated and often coexist in the same individual. There is an increasing evidence base linking an increased likelihood of cognitive dysfunction in subjects with diabetes especially of long duration. The assessment of cognitive function using standard cognitive screening tests is recommended in the routine assessment of all older people with diabetes.

Tips for Practice
- Clinicians must ensure that there is a major emphasis on quality of life and well-being for each older person with diabetes.

- Interventions must be planned early on in order to ensure their effectiveness.
- Practitioners should ensure there is a commitment to improve and/or *maintain* functional status.
- The presence of depressive symptoms must be ascertained, and clinical diagnosis of depression must be considered when evaluating cognitive function in older people with diabetes.

5.6   Conclusion

This chapter has considered some of the psychological issues for individuals in four special groups of people with diabetes. It is clear that there remain challenges in the care and treatment of minority ethnic groups and especially in the assessment of psychological well-being. Use of currently recommended screening tools for identifying depression in people with diabetes may be problematic, especially in minority ethnic groups, where the assessment tools used may not always be culturally appropriate. Recommendations for care for women with diabetes during pregnancy include an increased level of monitoring during pregnancy. However, although these recommendations are aimed at optimizing outcomes for women, they may have a negative psychological impact on the personal experience of pregnancy and childbirth. Therefore, appropriate support needs to be given at all stages of pregnancy and childbirth.

Diabetes is commonly associated with several comorbidities which can influence the treatment required, affect the outcome of any intervention, and alter health status and life quality. The often substantial increases in treatment, while improving the physical health status of the individual, can have a negative impact on psychological well-being. An awareness of this potential impact and the identification of patients in need of psychological support are vital in order to promote complete well-being. There are important implications for the care of older people with diabetes, where there may be high levels of medical comorbidity along with increased risk of depression and/or cognitive impairment. Distinguishing between these two latter categories is important in order to provide the most appropriate care.

Practice implications
- Recognizing and screening for depression is an important aspect of routine care for all people with diabetes; this can be more challenging in people from minority ethnic groups, in older people, and people with comorbidities.
- Person-centered care that takes account of the psychological impact of diabetes and other physical/medical comorbidities is essential and will be influenced by the special needs of the individual.

References

1. Bellary S, O'Hare JP, Raymond NT, Gumber A, Mughal S, Szczepura A, Kumer S, Barnett AH, for UKADS Study Group. Enhanced diabetes care to patients of south Asian ethnic origin (the United Kingdom Asian Diabetes Study): a cluster randomized controlled trial. Lancet. 2008;371:1769–76.
2. Holt RIG, Phillips DIW, Jameson KA, Cooper C, Dennison EM, Peveler RC. The relationship between depression and diabetes mellitus: findings from the Hertfordshire Cohort Study. Diabet Med. 2009;26:641–8.
3. Lloyd CE, Underwood L, Winkley K, Nouwen A, Hermanns N, Pouwer F. The epidemiology of diabetes and depression. In: Katon W, Maj M, Sartorius N, editors. Depression and diabetes. Chichester: Wiley/Blackwell; 2010.
4. Stone M, Lloyd CE. Psychological consequences of diabetes. In: Khunti K, Kumar S, Brodie J, editors. Diabetes UK and South Asian Health Foundation recommendations on diabetes research priorities for British South Asians. London: Diabetes UK; 2009.
5. Lloyd CE, Pambianco G, Orchard TJ. Does diabetes-related distress explain the presence of depressive symptoms and/or poor self-care in individuals with Type 1 diabetes? Diabet Med. 2010;27:234–7.
6. Asghar S, Hussain A, Ali S, Khan A, Magnusson A. Prevalence of depression and diabetes: a population-based study from rural Bangladesh. Diabet Med. 2007;24:872–7.

7. Zahid N, Asghar S, Claussen B, Hussain A. Depression and diabetes in a rural community in Pakistan. Diabetes Res Clin Pract. 2008; 79:124–7.

8. Mentality, for NIMHE: Guidelines for mental health promotion with black and minority ethnic communities. Mentality. http://www.be4researchproject.org.uk/BMEG%20Toolkit%20for%20Consultation.doc (2003). Accessed 29th November, 2011.

9. Department of Health. Positive steps. Supporting race equality in mental health care. London: Department of Health; 2007.

10. Bhui K, Bhugra D. Transcultural psychiatry: some social and epidemiological research issues. Int J Soc Psychiatry. 2001;47:1–9.

11. Diabetes UK. Minding the gap; the provision of psychological support and care for people with diabetes in the UK. London: Diabetes UK; 2008.

12. Arroll B, Khin N, Kerse N. Screening for depression in primary care with two verbally asked questions: cross sectional study. Br Med J. 2003;327:1144–6.

13. Whooley MA, de Jonge P, Vittinghoff E, Otte C, Moos R, Carney RM, Ali S, Dowray S, Na B, Feldman MD, Schiller NB, Browner WS. Depressive symptoms, health behaviors, and risk of cardiovascular events in patients with coronary heart disease. J Am Med Assoc. 2008;300:2379–88.

14. Spitzer RL, Kroenke K, Williams JB, the Patient Health Questionnaire Primary Care Study Group. Validation and utility of a self-report version of the PRIME-MD: the PHQ primary care study. JAMA. 1999;282:1737–44.

15. Williams R, Eley S, Hunt K, Bhatt S. Has psychological distress among UK South Asians been under-estimated? A comparison of three measures in the west of Scotland population. Ethn Health. 1997;2:21–9.

16. Lloyd CE, Sturt J, Johnson MRD, Mughal S, Collins G, Barnett AH. Development of alternative modes of data collection in South Asians with Type 2 diabetes. Diabet Med. 2008;25(4):455–62.

17. Bech P, Olsen LR, Kjoller M, Rasmussen NK. Measuring well-being rather than absence of distress symptoms: a comparison of the SF-36 Mental Health subscale and the WHO-Five Well-being scale. Int J Methods Psychiatr Res. 2003;12:85–91.

18. Henkel V, Mergl R, Kohnen R, Allgaier AK, Moller HJ, Hegerl U. Use of brief depression screening tools in primary care: consideration of heterogeneity in performance in different patient groups. Gen Hosp Psychiatry. 2004;26:190–8.

19. Lloyd CE, Johnson MRD, Mughal S, Sturt JA, Collins GS, Roy T, Bibi R, Barnett AH. Securing recruitment and obtaining informed consent in minority ethnic groups in the UK. BMC Health Serv Res. 2008;8:68.

20. Fagerli RA, Lien ME, Wandel M. Experience of dietary advice among Pakistani-born persons with type 2 diabetes in Oslo. Appetite. 2005;45:295–304.
21. Greenhalgh T, Helman C, Chowdhury AM. Health beliefs and folk models of diabetes in British Bangladeshis: a qualitative study. Br Med J. 1998;316:978–83.
22. Curtis S, Beirne J, Jude E. Advantages of training Asian diabetes support workers for Asian families and diabetes health care professionals. Pract Diabetes Int. 2003;20(6):215–8.
23. National Institute of Health and Clinical Excellence (NICE): Diabetes in pregnancy: management of diabetes and its complications from pre-conception to the post-natal period. Clinical guideline 63. London: NICE. Available at: http://www.nice.org.uk/nicemedia/live/11946/41320/41320.pdf(2008). Accessed 11 July 2011.
24. CEMACH. Confidential Enquiry into Maternal and Child Health. Diabetes in pregnancy: are we providing the best care? London: CEMACH; 2007.
25. Coulthard T, Hawthorne G, on behalf of the Northern Diabetes Pregnancy Service. Type 2 diabetes in pregnancy; more to come? Pract Diabetes Int. 2008;25(9):359–61.
26. Kim C, Sinco B, Kieffer EA. Racial and ethnic variation in access to health care; provision of health care services and ratings of health among women with histories of gestational diabetes mellitus. Diabetes Care. 2007;30:1459–65.
27. Katbamna S. Race and childbirth. Buckingham: Open University Press; 2000.
28. Murphy HR, Temple RC, Ball VE, et al. Personal experiences of women with diabetes who do not attend pre-pregnancy care. Diabet Med. 2010;27(1):92–100.
29. Lavender T, Platt MJ, Tsekiri E, Casson I, Byrom S, Nbaker L, Walkishaw S. Women's perceptions of being pregnancy and having pregestational diabetes. Midwifery. 2010;26:589–95.
30. CEMACH. Confidential Enquiry into Maternal and Child Health (CEMACH). Perinatal mortality 2008. London: CEMACH; 2010.
31. Barahona MJ, Sucunza N, Garcia-Patterson A, Hernandez M, Adelantado JM, Ginovart G, De Leiva A, Corcoy R. Period of gestational diabetes mellitus diagnosis and maternal and fetal morbidity. Acta Obstet Gynecol Scand. 2005;84(7):622–7.
32. Waddingham S: Looking after women with diabetes during pregnancy. Br J Prim Care Nurs;5. http://wwwbjpcn-cardiovascular.com/download/3086 (2008).
33. Crowther CA, Hiller JE, Moss JR, McPhee AJ, Jeffries WS, Robinson JS. Effect of treatment of gestational diabetes mellitus on pregnancy outcomes. N Engl J Med. 2005;352(24):247–2486.
34. Gabbe SG, Graves CR. Management of diabetes mellitus complicating pregnancy. Obstet Gynaecol. 2003;102(4):857–68.

35. Williams A, Modder J. Management of pregnancy complicated by diabetes-Maternal glycaemic control during pregnancy and neonatal management. Early Hum Dev. 2010;86(5):269–73.
36. Hildingsson I, Waldenstrom U, Radestad I. Women's expectations on antenatal care as assessed in early pregnancy: number of visits, continuity of caregiver and general content. Acta Obstet Gynecol Scand. 2002;81(2):118–25.
37. Robson SJ, Leader LR, Dear KBG, Bennett MJ. Women's expectations of management in their next pregnancy after an unexplained stillbirth: an internet-based empirical study. Aust N Z J Obstet Gynaecol. 2009;49:642–6.
38. Kim C, Newton K, Knopp RH. Gestational diabetes and incidence of type 2 diabetes mellitus: a systematic review. Diabetes Care. 2002;25:1862–8.
39. Ratner RE, Christophi CA, Metzger BE, Dabelea D, Bennett PH, Pi-Sunyer X, Fowler S, Kahn SE, the Diabetes Prevention Program Research Group. Prevention of diabetes in women with a history of gestational diabetes: effects of metformin and lifestyle interventions. J Clin Endocrinol Metab. 2008;93(12):4774–9.
40. Department of Health. National service framework for diabetes. London: Department of Health; 2001.
41. Anderson RM, Funnell MM. The art of empowerment. Alexandria: American Diabetes Association; 2001.
42. Diabetes UK: Diabetes in pregnancy notes. http://www.diabetes.org. uk/Professionals/Shared_Practice/Care_Topics/Pregnancy/ Diabetes-in-pregnancy-notes/ (2011). Accessed 1 Feb 2011.
43. Valderas JM, Starfield B, Sibbald B, Salisbury C, Roland M. Defining comorbidity: implications for understanding health and health services. Ann Fam Med. 2009;7(4):357–63.
44. Slater M, Perruccio AV, Badley EM. Musculoskeletal comorbidities in cardiovascular disease, diabetes and respiratory disease: the impact on activity limitations; a representative population-based study. BMC Public Health. 2011;11(1):77.
45. Zhao G, Ford ES, Balluz LS. Physical activity in U.S. older adults with diabetes mellitus: prevalence and correlates of meeting physical activity recommendations. J Am Geriatr Soc. 2011;59(1):132–7.
46. Prisciandaro JJ, Gebregziabher M, Grubaugh AL, Gilbert GE, Echols C, Egede LE. Impact of physical comorbidity on mortality in veterans with type 2 diabetes. Diabetes Technol Ther. 2011; 13(1):73–8.
47. Vitry AI, Roughhead EE, Preiss AK, et al. Influence of comorbidities on therapeutic progression of diabetes treatment in Australian veterans: a cohort study. PLoS One. 2010;5(11):e14024.
48. Charlson ME, Pompei P, Ales KL, MacKenzie CR. A new method of classifying prognostic comorbidity in longitudinal studies: development and validation. J Chronic Dis. 1987;40(5):373–83.

49. Fried LP, Tangen C, Walston J, et al. Frailty in older adults: evidence for a phenotype. J Gerontol. 2001;56A(3):M1–11.

50. Zeyfang A, Walston JD. Perspectives on diabetes care in old age: a focus on frailty. In: Sinclair AJ, editor. Diabetes in old age. 3rd ed. Chichester: Wiley; 2009.

51. Barzilay JI, Blaum C, Moore T, et al. Insulin resistance and inflammation as precursors of frailty: the Cardiovascular Health Study. Arch Intern Med. 2007;167(7):635–41.

52. Abdelhafiz AH. Coronary heart disease. In: Sinclair AJ, editor. Diabetes in old age. 3rd ed. Chichester: Wiley; 2009.

53. Haffner SM, Lehto S, Ronnemaa T, et al. Mortality from coronary heart disease in subjects with type 2 diabetes and in nondiabetic with and without prior myocardial infarction. N Engl J Med. 1998;339:229–34.

54. Morley JE, Sinclair A. The metabolic syndrome in older persons: a loosely defined constellation of symptoms or a distinct entity? Age Ageing. 2009;38(5):494–7.

55. Alexander CM, Landsman PB, Teutsch SM, et al. NCEP-defined metabolic syndrome, diabetes, and prevalence of coronary heart disease among NHANES III participants aged 50 years and older. Diabetes. 2003;52:1210–4.

56. Sinclair AJ. Diabetes in old age. In: Holt RIG, Cockram CS, Flyvbjerg A, Goldstein BJ, editors. Textbook of diabetes. 4th ed. Oxford: Wiley/Blackwell; 2010.

57. Gregg EW, Yaffe K, Cauley JA, Rolka DB, Blackwell TL, Narayan KM, Cummings SR. Is diabetes associated with cognitive impairment and cognitive decline among older women? Arch Intern Med. 2000;160:174–80.

58. Sinclair AJ, Girling AJ, Bayer AJ. Cognitive dysfunction in older subjects with diabetes mellitus: impact on diabetes self-management and use of care services: All Wales Research into Elderly (AWARE) study. Diabetes Res Clin Pract. 2000;50:203–12.

59. Munshi M, Grande L, Hayes M, Ayres D, Suhl E, Capelson R, Lins S, Milberg W, Weinger K. Cognitive dysfunction is associated with poor diabetes control in older adults. Diabetes Care. 2006;29: 1794–9; 56:42–8.

60. Cukierman T, Gerstein HC, et al. Cognitive decline and dementia in diabetes–systematic overview of prospective observational studies. Diabetologia. 2005;48(12):2460–9.

61. Amato L, Paolisso G, Cacciatore F, Ferrara N, Canonico S, Rengo F, Varricchio M. Non-insulin-dependent diabetes mellitus is associated with a greater prevalence of depression in the elderly. The Osservatorio Geriatrico of Campania Region Group. Diabetes Metab. 1996;22(5):314–8.

62. Anderson RJ, Freedland KE, Clouse RE, Lustman PJ. The prevalence of co-morbid depression in adults with diabetes. Diabetes Care. 2001;6:1069–78.
63. Lustman PJ, Anderson RJ, Freedland KE, De Groot M, Carney RM, Clouse RE. Depression and poor glycemic control. A meta-analytic review of the literature. Diabetes Care. 2000;23:934–42.
64. Egede LE, Zheng D, Simpson K. Comorbid depression is associated with increased health care use and expenditures in individuals with diabetes. Diabetes Care. 2002;25(3):464–70.
65. Sinclair AJ, Asimakopoulou K. Diabetes and cognitive dysfunction. In: Sinclair AJ, editor. Diabetes in old age. 3rd ed. Chichester: Wiley; 2009.

Chapter 6
Tips and Tricks on Effective Communication with People with Diabetes: Helping People Achieve Their Goals While Achieving Your Own

Sue Cradock and Katharine D. Barnard

6.1 Introduction

The aim of this chapter is to help the reader consider their approach as a key component of behavior change in people with diabetes. We may all believe that this is a key aspect of our role, but how many of us ask ourselves:

"What am I doing wrong?"
"Why will my patients not take notice of me?"

S. Cradock (✉)
Department of Health and Sciences,
University of Leicester, Hampshire,
England

K.D. Barnard
Faculty of Medicine, University of Southampton,
Enterprise Road, Southampton Science Park, Chilworth,
Southampton, SO16 7NS, UK
e-mail: k.barnard@soton.ac.uk

K.D. Barnard and C.E. Lloyd (eds.), *Psychology and Diabetes Care*,   135
DOI 10.1007/978-0-85729-573-6_6,
© Springer-Verlag London Limited 2012

> "Why do people seem to want to change their lifestyle when we talk about it but come back not having made any changes?"

These questions (and many more that you are asking yourself) may give a signal of our frustration, which for some healthcare professions leads to being distanced and judgmental:

A lot of patients tell us that they exercise and eat well and are living a perfect life, and wonder why their [blood sugar] values are so high. It's at that moment that our problems become obvious. We can't counter their claim with anything because we know they're not telling us the truth [1].

For others, it leads to a sense of not being able to do the job well or not being in control:

At the first meeting, I want to inform the patient somewhat, but a lot of patients are one step ahead…and are really treading on my toes. They want to learn about self-tests and want to prick their fingers and, at that moment, I feel that the discussion has taken a wrong turn. It is wrong to me…but, on the other hand, they maybe want to do something practical, and don't have enough energy to listen to all the information…it is normal for nurses to feel like this…I mean, [to feel] that the consultation has gone wrong [1]

These experiences are now recognized as a result of a possible clash of "cultures" or paradigms [2]. Healthcare professionals are trained to provide "acute care" which is characterized by the patient bringing a problem into the consulting room and the healthcare professional taking a history, making a diagnosis, and prescribing treatment (which may involve lifestyle changes). This approach appears to work well when the patient is unwell and so is motivated to "take the advice" in the short term to aid their recovery. The challenge to this comes when the patient feels well; the prescribed changes are numerous, are required to be followed for life, impact on most aspects of daily life (food, physical activity, spontaneity); and the promise of benefit of these changes are in the future…not now!

Chapters 1 and 2 have outlined how living with diabetes can be hard work. The immediate demands of adjusting to the diagnosis and subsequent lifestyle changes combined with the changing attitudes of other people contribute to the challenge of having diabetes. Rather than a "fix it" pill from the doctor, the role of healthcare professionals is to provide expert advice and support self-management and help people make sometimes significant lifestyle behavior changes.

This chapter is designed to help you reflect on your own practice, on why you do what you do, what the impact is of what you do and provide some tips to help you change what you are doing, should you wish to do so. We aim to do this by providing some insights that we have gained in relation to working with people with diabetes and understanding how changing the way that we work could have an impact on the way that your "patients" work with themselves and their own diabetes.

6.1.1   A Moment for Reflection

For you to reflect on your own work as we go along, we believe it is worth spending a moment before reading on to consider the nature of your current work with people with diabetes by considering the following questions:

1. What do you believe the purpose of your role is?
2. What makes a consultation successful for you?
3. What do you imagine makes a consultation successful for your patients?
4. What makes a consultation a failure for you?
5. What do you imagine makes a consultation a failure for your patients?
6. What frustrates you most about your work with people with diabetes?
7. What would you most like to change about your work that will help you deliver better care to people with diabetes?

Please see Springer Extra Materials (http://extras.springer. com/) for a worksheet to use while exploring your thoughts on current practice.

6.2   What People Believe Drives What They Do

To help people change their current behaviors, it may be of value to help them explore their beliefs and perceptions about their diabetes and its effects. Psychology research has now clearly shown that when people develop a long-term health condition (e.g., diabetes), they will have a number of questions that they ask – which can be summarized as follows:

- What is the cause?
- What is it?
- How long will it last?
- How will it affect me?
- What can I do about it?

And that their personal answers to these questions will have a direct impact on their levels of self-care. These beliefs have also been shown to be predictive of overall mortality, morbidity, and diabetes complications [13]. One name for this model is the "commonsense model" but is also known as the Illness Perceptions Model or the Self-Regulatory Model [3]. This model has been used to show that helping people with diabetes reflect on their own beliefs in relation to diabetes is now recognized as important in supporting behavior change to support self-care [3–9].

Depending on how people respond to these questions, this will inform what they do to take care of themselves. Our beliefs drive our behaviors.

Case Study
Consider Anne, who is 48 and was diagnosed with type 2 diabetes 6 months ago. When she was diagnosed by her GP, she was advised, "Don't worry, it is not serious, you do not need insulin." Add this to the fact that she feels reasonably well and was diagnosed by a routine

well-woman check. She is seeking to believe that she is ok and does not need to change much in her life (which is a busy one), so she may seek solace in her doctor's words and believe that "this is not serious." This belief then may drive a reduced motivation to make changes in her lifestyle.

Case Study

Consider Graham, who is 65 and has had type 2 diabetes for 10 years. He regularly attends his surgery for check-ups but struggles to change his day-to-day lifestyle. When challenged, he defends himself by saying that he goes to all his checkups and takes his medication – so he is trying! What do you think his underlying beliefs are that are preventing him from considering taking action?

Without exploring this with him, we cannot be sure, but consider what would make him defend his actions… that he is doing his best…perhaps believing that you are not? Or perhaps that he cannot do anything more?

Case Study

Liz, aged 57, believes she has had type 2 diabetes for a few years despite being diagnosed with it less than a year ago. She has been struggling with her weight for many years (her BMI is currently 37) and now feels that her diabetes is related to that, that she is responsible and that as she has not been able to reduce her weight, is resigned to the fact that, "nothing I do now can change anything." She believes she is powerless to change anything.

A man hears what he wants to hear and disbelieves the rest.
Simon and Garfunkel

We all keep hold onto beliefs that help us to continue to do what we want to do… and sometimes it is because we have never been given the chance to reflect on what we believe.

Consider for a moment, what reasons you give yourself for all/any/some of the following:

- Not following the speed limit when you are driving your car (when there is good evidence as to why you should)
- Not following the diet that you are advised
- Not following the physical activity levels that are advised
- Using your mobile phone when driving
- Drinking more alcohol than the recommendations advise

We suspect that, like us, you will find reasons to support your behaviors!

We have learned that spending time getting people with diabetes to "tell their story" about their diabetes may assist them in exploring their beliefs and possibly help them see what the barriers are for themselves in making changes. Many group education self-management programs use this approach [10], and the same can be used during consultations [11, 12]:

- What do you believe could be the effects of diabetes on you/your body?
- What do you believe could help prevent this?
- Who do you believe is the person most able to influence this?

Using an approach outlined in Chap. 6 will help you use these questions above.

6.3   Recognize Who Is in Control

People are usually doing what is right for them given their perception of the situation at the time. Their perception may be influenced by their health beliefs (see above), by insufficient/inaccurate knowledge, by the demands of their social situation, or by other factors.

So, someone who is not following the advice that you have given them will have good reasons – they have decided, for one reason or another, that it is not right for them. And as human beings, that is our right! But this is challenging when we, as healthcare professionals, cannot quite understand why people seem to not want to "take care of themselves." They are doing so, but in the way that they believe to be right for them. This is recognized in the concept of "empowerment" [13].

Anderson and Funnell [13] identified the fundamental principles of empowerment as being:

1. People with diabetes provide at least 98% of their own diabetes care, so we are limited in what we can help with!
2. The greatest impact on the patient's health and well-being is as a result of their self-management decisions/actions during the routine conduct of their daily life.
3. Diabetes is so woven into the fabric of the patient's life that many, if not most, of the routines of daily living affect and are affected by diabetes and its self-management.
4. Because patients are in control of their daily self-management decisions, they are responsible for those decision and the resulting consequences.
5. Patients cannot surrender the control or responsibility they have for diabetes self-management no matter how much they wish to do so. Even if patients turn their self-management completely over to a HCP, they can change their mind about that at any time. Thus, they remain in control at all times.
6. Healthcare professionals (HCPs)cannot control and therefore cannot be responsible for the self-care decisions of their patients
7. HCPs are responsible for doing all they can to ensure their patients are making informed self-management decisions, i.e., informed by an adequate understanding of diabetes self-management and an awareness of the aspects of their personal lives that influence their self-management decisions, and the potential impact of the decisions they make.

While empowerment has become a buzzword, exploring its real meaning fundamentally changed the practice of one of us, such that the work we undertook with people with diabetes changed because of one simple realization: that the person in the consulting room is an adult, is responsible for their own self-management, and has greater understanding of their own life that I do. So instead of behaving as if they were in a "child" role and the HCP taking on a "parent role," the roles became one of adult talking to adult. We stopped telling people what they should do (however nicely and however much they wanted us to – more of that later) and started exploring how they lived with diabetes, what were they most concerned about, what did they want to change, and how could they start going about doing that?

Let us reconsider Graham. It would be easy to make assumptions about his views about his diabetes care, but doing this may take us up a "garden path" and waste time; a good place to start opening up the conversation would be: what frustrates you most about your diabetes Graham? His immediate response may be "nothing…you are the ones that are worried," but the fact that he attends all of his appointments suggests that he has a level of concern, so perhaps, the next step for us would be to explore why he thinks we might be worried? This opens up a discussion about complications: helping us know that he is clear about this aspect of diabetes (note that it is a discussion not a teaching session, you are interested in what he actually knows NOT what he should know, and how the "medical checks" relate to the complications). Let us assume Graham knows all about the complications (as many people do) but that he seems to focus on "I can't make the changes you want me to." Rather than moving to justify the recommended changes, seek to understand what maybe the barriers for Graham to make changes. Using "curious" questions such as "what changes are the most difficult for you?" or "what changes have you been able to make?" or "what changes would you most want to make?," this helps you develop the conversation about change but with Graham setting the agenda – you are following the lead from his responses and not imposing your own.

6.4 Recognize the Power and Limitations of Your Role

There is a certain amount of power associated with the role of healthcare professionals, inherently woven into the socially constructed nature of hierarchical healthcare systems. Historically, the healthcare system has been based on the belief that healthcare professionals have the expertise and knowledge, which they impart to "patients" to tell them what they need to do, or take if a medication is prescribed, so that they can get better.

The management of chronic conditions such as diabetes, however, does not fit neatly within this paradigm for a number of reasons. Diabetes has no currently known cure; therefore, "patients" will never "get better"; healthcare professionals may have enormous knowledge and advice to give; however only people living with diabetes know whether they can or will incorporate that advice into their daily self-management routines; life is dynamic and new, often unexpected challenges crop up which impact to varying degrees on a person's ability to self-manage, irrespective of their best intentions.

With this reality in mind, it is important to recognize the crucial role that healthcare professionals have in supporting people with diabetes to optimize their diabetes control and quality of life. Indeed their role is crucial as they have direct contact with people with diabetes, and in the main, people take notice of them! This can be done following these simple principles:

- Recognize the limitations in telling people what to do – despite them wanting you to do so. We all want a quick fix to complex problems – we all would like other people to do the hard work! So explore why they want you to do that.
- Helping people explore themselves and what they want for their health.
- Helping people realize their responsibility.
- Helping people learn – which is different to teaching!
- Let go of the need to be responsible for the patient's outcomes...this is a pointless and futile exercise as there are so many factors that impact on patient outcomes.

- Be responsible for the processes (that influence outcomes) that you have control over! The way you ask questions, the way you respond to questions, the way you help people learn, the way you communicate risk, the way you help people think about what they are doing, and the way you support people to change what they want to change.
- Recognize what you can be responsible for helping them be clear about what they are doing, the impact, and what they want to change.

6.5   Recognize the Unleashed Power in the Patient

One of the key roles that we can play in helping someone with diabetes (or any long-term condition) is to help them realize what they are able to do. Many people have been "ground down" by the system of healthcare that expects them to make many (often unrealistic) changes to "help" control their diabetes. Many people attempt these changes, and some of course succeed. But for those that do not, a sense of help-lessness and of being a failure may develop. These states are likely to hinder any small changes that could make a big dif-ference in the future.

Case Study

Take Graham, 65 year old with type 2 diabetes. Graham is engaged in his diabetes care and regularly attends all scheduled medical appointments. On diagnosis, 10 years ago, Graham went on a strict diet and tried very hard to start a healthy exercise regimen. After a number of false starts and ambitious weight loss targets that he was unable to achieve, Graham became overwhelmed by the enormity of the lifestyle changes. Combined with this was his perceived disappointment that he felt from his doctor and nurse and his underlying feeling that they thought he was not trying hard enough.

With realistic goals and a stepped plan to achieve them, Graham could focus on smaller targets that would be more achievable and increase his self-confidence.

Self (or autonomous) motivation is the ability to motivate yourself, to find a reason and the necessary strength to do something, without the need of being influenced to do so by another person. Many of your patients will be motivated by you to change something, they will want to make themselves better, they will want to follow your instructions, and some will be motivated because they want to please you. If your patients are motivated by you to change something then the change is likely to be short lived as it is a change that is being imposed and so is not "internally" motivated. This has been described as "controlled" motivation, which may have roots in guilty feelings or external pressure from clinicians or family, (and) is unlikely to have lasting effects [14].

A good place to start to support "autonomous motivation" is by asking people what they want to change. This avoids imposing change and avoids focusing on what you want them to change. As their motivation and confidence to change builds, then they may naturally focus on the areas that you are most concerned about, but remember, some people may not – and of course, they have the right not to change!

Some diabetes researchers have developed "self-determination theory" (SDT) into a guided approach to be used by healthcare professions called guided self-determination. This aims to increase the patients' life skills, defined as "those personal, social, cognitive and physical skills that enable people to control and direct their lives, and to develop the capacity to live with and produce change in their environment" [15]. The method was developed to guide both patients with persistent poor glycemic control and the professionals working alongside them through mutual reflection drawing on a large number of semistructured worksheets and has been shown to improve outcomes for people with type 1 diabetes. Other researchers have studied the potential of healthcare professionals to support autonomous motivation in people with diabetes in a primary care setting and have concluded that, "training clinicians to increase their support of patient autonomy may be one important avenue to improve diabetes outcomes" [16]. A recent study suggested that because people living with diabetes "have difficulties maintaining multiple self-care demands," using SDT to guide consultations can support their efforts in "engaging patients in exploration of their motivations for making lifestyle changes" [17].

One way of supporting "positive" self-talk is by helping people see what they are "succeeding" at. Start by asking them "what do you think you are doing that helps manage your diabetes?" This may be:

- Taking their tablets regularly
- Managing to maintain their weight
- Giving up/reducing smoking
- Changing something in their diet

Follow this up with exploring what they are most concerned about and how they would like this to change: this will start to unleash the power of self-motivation. We are all motivated to do exactly what we are doing now! But just occasionally, someone asking us to explore that will uncover something we want to change, and then we can start working on that!

Case Study

Anne, 48 years old and diagnosed with type 2 diabetes 6 months ago. On diagnosis by her GP, Anne was advised, "Don't worry, it is not serious, you do not need insulin"; however this combined with not feeling particularly ill has led Anne to believe her condition is not serious. With an already busy lifestyle, Anne does not realize the progressive nature of type 2 diabetes and the importance of making positive, achievable lifestyle changes now to delay the risk of diabetes-related complications in the future.

A starting point with Anne is maybe to ask her what she is most concerned about when she thinks about her diabetes. Her response will then guide you to the next question:

If she answers "nothing," then this may prompt you to be curious as to why that is?

Most likely (in the experience of one of us), she will respond with something like:

"Well of course I know it can be serious, but I am ok."

This may prompt you to ask, "What would it take for you to believe it was serious?" Her responses would then provide you with information to help provide Anne with information that may help her rethink.

Note that this approach does not start with telling her what can go wrong...but starts with what she believes.

Another positive avenue is to focus on rewarding "effort" rather than outcome. Many variables influence outcomes, and for people to feel motivated, they need to feel a sense of accomplishment even when they are not achieving the outcome they want. Even more effective is when the "reward" or "praise" comes from the individual themselves rather than you. Turn "Oh well done, you should be proud of that" (telling people what they should be feeling) into "And how do you feel about what you have achieved?"

A word of caution is to avoid using "failure" words; you may be talking about "tablet failure," but the person in front of you may be thinking they are failing. And of course if they do think it is the tablet "failing," then they may stop taking them!

The use of phrases such as "tablet failure" and "failed on diet and exercise" implies that success is possible. Yet we know that glycemia control will deteriorate over time, and the requirement for additional therapy is to be expected, and not a sign of failure. You may need to explore what "success" means to your patients as they may think success is about not getting worse, and of course, this is not true in type 2 diabetes.

> **Case Study**
> Take Graham again. Graham believes he has made gargantuan efforts to improve his lifestyle but has "failed" to slow the progression of his diabetes. The advice from his GP to lose two and a half stones has succeeded only in contributing to Graham's already deepening sense of helplessness and conviction that any attempt to lose weight will result in a similar way to all previous attempts, in failure.

6.6   Use Tips and Tools to Help You Share the Responsibility

6.6.1   Focus on the Small Things

Small things can often mean "big barriers," and while something may seem trivial and almost like an excuse for inaction to a third party, for the individual, it may not seem at all "small." Focusing on the context of behavior change, what it looks like in daily life and how it could fit without too much inconvenience or readjustment to routines can be very useful in helping people understand the achievability of making that change as well as the potential benefits of success.

6.6.2   Use Something to Draw/Write/Explore on (Rollnick and Zoffmann Tools): Let the Patient Do the Writing!

It does not have to be a whizzy computer tool to be useful; often one of the most effective ways to explore the barriers and benefits of making a behavior change is to write down all the (alternative methods may be required for those who cannot write) information on a piece of paper. Something as basic as the example in Table 6.1 can be a useful start in opening up a discussion around the steps needed to make a behavior change and how to tackle the barriers to achieving it. This is explored in greater detail in Chap. 7.

TABLE 6.1   Goal setting worksheet

What is the goal?	Why is it important?	How will you achieve it?	What will stop you?	How will you overcome this barrier?

6.6.3   Learn to Manage Silence

It is very tempting, almost irresistible, to jump into a gap in the conversation and fill it with "helpful advice." People need time to consider the information they have just been given or how to answer a question asked. If the answer came quickly, then it is unlikely you would be discussing the behavior change in question as it would already have been achieved. Different people use different techniques to stop them "filling the silence" such as counting backward in their head or reciting nursery rhymes in their head. Supporting people to self-manage their diabetes means giving them space to find solutions that will work for them.

6.6.4   Keep a List of "Open Discovery" Questions Nearby as a Prompt

It can be difficult to think of the "right" question to ask that will open up discussion and enable someone to really explore their beliefs and reasons for actions. Keeping a short list of "open discovery" questions nearby can be a helpful prompt to ask an appropriate question at the right time. Questions such as:

- What frustrates you most about your diabetes?
- What makes you think that?
- What do you think would happen if …?
- How could you change that?
- How would you feel if you were able to achieve that?

6.6.5   Ask the Patient What Their Issues Are Before Introducing Yours

During busy clinics, with targets to achieve and tasks that must be done within a limited amount of time, be honest with your patient about what your agenda is but also ask them for their agenda ("What do you most want to achieve in the next 10–15 min?"). You have started the conversation by being clear about what time you have and what you have to achieve, but you have also demonstrated that you recognize that there are two people in the conversation, both of whom may have conflicting needs of the available time! What makes a consultation valuable to the healthcare professional may not make it valuable to the patient.

6.6.6   Finish All Consultations with a Time of Reflection for You and Them

The last few minutes of the consultation can often be the most important in the desire for behavior change! Using it to reflect on what has been discussed and being clear about goals set will help people walk away from the consultation with a greater chance of success. This can be facilitated by the use of a sheet of paper that the patient uses to make notes on in the absence of a purpose designed "care plan." Encouraging the patient to write is more likely to make the paper "plan" be read again and used!

Example
What is my personal goal from today?
....
....
What will I do to achieve this goal?
....
....
Check progress every week and review.
....
....

6.6.7   If You Find that You Keep Running Out of Time…

Try to avoid this by being clear about how much time you have to start with, keep a clock close by so that you both see how the time is going. This approach will help both you and your patient be reminded about what time is left.

Try to avoid going into "information giving" overload in the hope that "something will go in" and "I will have done my job." If you need to make sure that you provided certain key bits of information, then having this ready, in written form, may enable you to use whatever time you have left more effectively. This "list" could be made potentially more effective by leaving spaces for the patient to make comments by … and therefore to personalize.

6.7   Do Not Get Hung Up on the Theory

There are many theories/models/approaches in the literature; we have mentioned some throughout this chapter and another couple that are often considered in healthcare are discussed below.

6.7.1   Motivational Interviewing

Motivational interviewing is a client-centered, directive method for enhancing intrinsic motivation to change by exploring and resolving ambivalence, which has been found effective [18]. It recognizes and accepts the fact that clients who need to make changes in their lives approach such changes at different levels of readiness to change their behavior. It is nonjudgmental and nonconfrontational. The approach aims? To increase the individual's awareness of the potential problems caused, consequences experienced, and risks faced as a result of the behavior in question. Alternatively, healthcare professionals help individuals envisage a better future, and the individuals become increasingly motivated to achieve it. Either way, the strategy seeks to help clients think differently about their behavior and ultimately to consider what might be gained through change.

Motivational interviewing can be individual or group-based and is an increasingly popular and effective way to facilitate behavior change for people with diabetes [18].

6.7.2   Stages of Change/Transtheoretical Model of Behavior Change

This model is based on the premise that change occurs via a process of progress involving a number of stages. These stages are:

- Precontemplation – the individual is unaware that their behavior is problematic and does not consider behavior change to be necessary.
- Contemplation – the individual is starting to recognize that their behavior is problematic and is considering the benefits and downsides of that behavior.
- Preparation – the individual is intending to take action in the immediate future and may begin taking small steps toward change.
- Action – the individual has made specific changes to their behavior, and positive change has occurred.
- Maintenance – the individual is working to maintain the behavior change and prevent relapse.
- Termination – the individual is confident they can continue the behavior change and will not return to their old unhealthy behavior [19].

A criticism of this model has been that it is not possible to know for sure which stage an individual is in and therefore how best to help move them on to the next stage [20].

Overall, these approaches give us a clearer understanding of the mechanisms underlying people's thinking in relation to behavior change and health beliefs. There is, however, no "magic bullet" that will enable your patients to change their behavior in the way that you want them to. All of the approaches that are shown to have an impact involve the healthcare professional changing their approach ... so to change the way your patients behave, you may have to start with yourself!

But, as we have already suggested, behavior change can be hard for many of us, and researchers have shown that while healthcare professionals wished to change their practice, that training alone was not enough to help most people change their approach [2, 21]. We have found the following to be helpful when trying to change our approach to consultations:

1. Be clear about what you are already doing and what you want to change. One of us has regularly videoed/audio-taped their work to actually see what they were doing.
2. Explore your personal motivation for change – what would help you? What do you expect to be different as a result?
3. Develop a clear plan of what you want to change first.
4. Make time in your work for the reflection/planning to take place. At least 2 hours!
5. Use trusted colleagues to help you with feedback but make sure they know what you want feedback on! We usually need another person to see what we are doing well, rather than what we could improve...we tend to easily see what needs to change!

References

1. Hornsten A, Lundman B, Almberg A, Sandstrom H. Nurses experiences of conflicting encounters in diabetes care. Eur Diabetes Nurs. 2008;5(2):64–9.
2. Anderson RM, Funnell MM. Patient Empowerment: reflections on the challenge of fostering the adoption of a new paradigm. Patient Educ Couns. 2005;57:153–7.
3. Hagger MS, Orbell S. A meta-analytic review of the common-sense model of illness representations. Psychol Health. 2003;18(2): 141–84.
4. Skinner T, Carey M, Cradock S, Daly H, Davies M, Doherty Y, Heller S, Khunti K, Oliver L. Diabetes education and self-management for ongoing and newly diagnosed (DESMOND): process modelling of pilot study. Patient Educ Couns. 2006;64(1):369–77.
5. McAndrew LM, Musumeci-Szabó TJ, Mora PA, Vileikyte L, Burns E, Halm EA, Leventhal EA, Leventhal H. Using the common sense

model to design interventions for the prevention and management of chronic illness threats: from description to process. Br J Health Psychol. 2008;13:195–204.

6. Leventhal H, Diefenbach M, Leventhal EA. Illness cognition: using common sense to understand treatment adherence and affect cognition interactions. Cog Ther Res. 1992;162:143–63.

7. Weinehall L, Johnson O, Jansson JH, Boman K, Huhtasaari F, Hallmans G, Dahlen GH, Wall S. Perceived health modifies the effect of biomedical risk factors in the prediction of acute myocardial infarction: an incident case–control study from northern Sweden. J Intern Med. 1998;243:99–107.

8. Idler EL, Benyamini Y. Self-rated health and mortality: a review of twenty-seven community studies. J Health Soc Behav. 1997; 38:21–37.

9. Hayes AJ, Clarke PM, Glasziou PG, Simes RJ, Drury PL, Keech AC. Can self-rated health scores be used for risk prediction in patients with type 2 diabetes? Diabetes Care. 2008;31:795–7.

10. Davies MJ, Heller S, Skinner TC, Campbell MJ, Carey ME, Cradock S, Dallosso HM, Daly H, Doherty Y, Eaton S, Fox C, Oliver L, Rantell K, Rayman G, Khunti K, on behalf of the DESMOND Collaborative. Effectiveness of the diabetes education and self-management for ongoing and newly diagnosed (DESMOND) programme for people with newly diagnosed type 2 diabetes: cluster randomised controlled trial. Br Med J. 2008;336:491–5.

11. Skinner TC, Cradock S, Barnard KD, Parkin T. Patient & professional accuracy of recalled treatment decisions in outpatient consultations. Diabet Med. 2007;24:557–60.

12. Latter S, Sibley A, Skinner TC, Cradock S, Zinken KM, Lussier MT, Richard C, Roberge D. The impact of an intervention for nurse prescribers on consultations to promote patient medicine-taking in diabetes: a mixed methods study. Int J Nurs Stud. 2010;47(9):1126–38.

13. Anderson RM, Funnell MM. Patient empowerment: myths and misconceptions. Patient Educ Couns. 2010;79:277–82.

14. Zoffmann V: Guided self-determination: a life skills approach developed in difficult type 1 diabetes. PhD thesis. Department of nursing science, University of Aarhus, Aarhus; 2004.

15. Zoffmann V, Lauritzen T. Guided self-determination improves life skills with Type 1 diabetes and A1C in randomized controlled trial. Patient Educ Couns. 2006;64:78–86.

16. Shigaki C, et al. Motivation and diabetes self-management. Chronic Illn. 2010;6:202–14.

17. Williams GC, et al. Variation in perceived competence, glycemic control, and patient satisfaction: relationship to autonomy support from physicians. Patient Educ Couns. 2005;57:39–45.

18. Rollnick S, Mason P, Butler C. Health behaviour change: a guide for practitioners. Edinburgh: Churchill Livingstone; 1999.

19. Prochaska JO, DiClemente CC, Norcross JC. In search of how people change. Applications to addictive behaviors. Am Psychol. 1992;47(9):1102–14.
20. Littell JH, Girvin H. Stages of change. A critique. Behav Modif. 2002;26:223–73.
21. Pill R, Rees ME, Stott NCH, Rollnick SR. Can nurses let go? Issues arising from an intervention designed to improve patients' involvement with their own care. J Adv Nurs. 1999;6:1492–9.

Chapter 7
Supporting Health Behavior Change in General Practice

Colin Greaves

Previous chapters have emphasized the importance of using a patient-centered communication style and have presented some useful techniques for helping people to plan and learn how to succeed in making changes in lifestyle behavior. This chapter aims to reinforce and build on these ideas to understand clearly *how* behavior change works and how to support lifestyle change in a busy practice setting.

7.1 Share the Power

Patients will only make changes if *they* decide that it is something that they want to do. Adopting a patient-centered style and using the techniques for active patient involvement described in Chap. 6 will help to get your patients ready for change. However, getting motivated is only the first step!

C. Greaves
Peninsula College of Medicine and Dentistry, University of Exeter,
Magdalen Road, Exeter, Devon EX1 2LU, UK
e-mail: colin.greaves@pms.ac.uk

K.D. Barnard and C.E. Lloyd (eds.), *Psychology and Diabetes Care*,   157
DOI 10.1007/978-0-85729-573-6_7,
© Springer-Verlag London Limited 2012

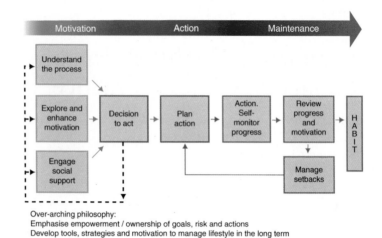

FIGURE 7.1 The process model of lifestyle behavior change (Greaves et al. [3])

7.2   Have a Plan

Having an idea in your mind about the way in which behavior change works is extremely useful to help you decide what to do next with the patient in front of you. If you know where they are on the journey, you can more easily decide what you need to do to move them forward. Figure 7.1 is a diagram of how behavior change works. This presents behavior change as a journey in three stages and was developed from a wide-ranging review of scientific evidence about what intervention components were associated with success in interventions to change diet or increase physical activity [1]. It also formed the basis for a Diabetes Prevention Toolkit offered alongside a recent European diabetes prevention guideline [2].

Essentially, there are three stages on the journey of behavior change: getting motivated, planning action, and keeping going. Each of these stages requires a different focus for providing support. So, if you know where your patient is on this journey, this helps you to decide what to do to help them take the next step. The following text explains the model in more

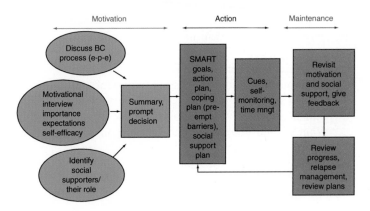

FIGURE 7.2 Techniques for supporting behavior change

detail and gives some hints about what kind of techniques you might use, depending what stage your patient is at (and see Fig. 7.2 also for a summary). The choice of techniques may vary of course, depending on the resources available and the individual patient.

Although developed for supporting changes in diet and physical activity, the same processes are likely to apply to stopping smoking, managing alcohol intake, and adhering to diabetes medication.

7.2.1 Understanding the Process of Behavior Change

Each individual should be able to understand the basic process of behavior change, including likely challenges and what kind of support might help them to achieve success. A key piece of information to get across is that making a change is not simply a case of deciding what to do and then going out to do it. Changing behavior is a journey, and it takes time to break down old habits and replace them with new ones. You will encounter obstacles and setbacks along the way, so you will need a strong, clear motivation and careful planning – you would not set out on a long journey without having a clear idea where you wanted to go or without a map or a plan of how to get there and changing your lifestyle is no different.

Possible behavior change techniques

- Ask about and build on existing experiences of behavior change (e.g. "have you ever tried to lose weight before? What happened?" "What do you think went wrong?" or "What helped you to succeed before you put the weight back on?").
- Building experience by trial and error (e.g. a small experiment to change one simple behavior over the next week) with subsequent discussion of what helped or prevented the patient from succeeding.
- Empowering information-exchange techniques, such as reflective listening (see Chap. 6) and using the elicit-provide-elicit (e-p-e) technique [4]. Essentially, this is an active learning approach which involves encouraging clients to first discuss their existing knowledge/experience (elicit), then supplying new information (provide), followed by further discussion (the second "elicit") to check they have understood fully and encouraging them to process the new material in relation to their own existing knowledge. This technique is also known more simply as "Ask, Tell, Discuss."
- Presenting information in the form of metaphors or stories (e.g. "behavior change is a journey, with many challenges and pitfalls along the way, but with good planning and strong motivation you will have the tools you need to find your way").

7.2.2 Exploring and Enhancing Motivation

Motivation consists of two important components: importance (having a good reason for making the change) and confidence (believing that you can do it!).

1. Importance: Patients should be able to weigh up the pros and cons of changing their diet and/or physical activity and decide if (on balance) it is important to make some

changes. Intervention strategies should aim to enhance perceived importance by focusing, for instance, on awareness of risk (how high is my risk of diabetes complications/ other health consequences?), and expectations of benefit (what effect will changing my behavior have on my diabetes control?).

Possible behavior change techniques
- Motivational interviewing (MI) techniques and other effective communication techniques (Chap. 6) [4].
- Decision balance tools (basically a line down the middle of a piece of paper inviting people to write down the pros and cons of making a change)
- Using communication techniques (as above: reflective listening; Ask, Tell, Discuss) to provide realistic and accurate information on risks and expectations

2. Confidence (self-efficacy): participants should develop the confidence to be able to carry out changes in their behavior.

Possible behavior change techniques
- Motivational interviewing techniques (e.g. questioning to determine key barriers and strengths for the individual patient).
- Setting goals in "small steps" to encourage confidence building over time.
- Identify likely barriers or problems and possible solutions (problem-solving). Using a "Confidence Ruler" can be a good way to explore confidence about making any specific behavior change (ask "on a scale of one to ten, how confident are you that you can …", then use their score to explore further "what is stopping this form being 2 points higher?" "what would it take to make this a 7 or 8?" etc.).
- Reinforce personal strengths and resources.

7.2.3   Engage Social Support

Each individual should be able to recognize the value of engaging friends or family in supporting attempts to change and be able to identify the type support that would be useful to him/her. A supporter can help in any of three ways:

- Practical support (e.g. giving lifts, buying or lending equipment, cooking meals, buying the right foods)
- Emotional support (e.g. making changes alongside the patient, being interested in her/his progress, being someone to talk to, offering encouragement or positive reinforcement)
- Informational support (e.g. helping to plan changes, or to find relevant information)

Evidence shows that involving social support (usually from a family member) as part of a weight loss intervention adds around 3 kg on average to the amount of weight loss achieved [5]. That is a pretty big deal, especially as it hardly costs you any time or effort!

Possible behavior change techniques
- Discuss with the patient (using communication skills as in Chap. 6) the pros and cons of getting a supporter involved. You can use the elicit-provide-elicit method again here (as above).
- Provide general information about the different types of social support (practical, emotional, informational).
- Encourage the patient to make social support part of her/his action plan (see below).
- Invite the supporter to attend any future discussions (or intervention sessions if you are running a group-based intervention).

7.2.4   Deciding to Act

This is basically about bringing the patient to the point of making a decision. Having discussed all the motivation-enhancing aspects above, you (and the patient) should now be able to summarize the advantages and disadvantages for the patient (from her/his point of view) of engaging in different behaviors.

The patient should be able to use this information to make a decision about whether or not to make some changes.

Possible behavior change techniques
- Summarize the patient's motivations and reasons for confidence you have discussed so far, acknowledging the main barriers to change and the patient's ideas/any discussions you have had about how these might be overcome.
- Ask an open-ended question to prompt the patient to make a decision. For instance, asking "so where does that leave you?" is a nice way to really put the ball in the patient's court.

7.2.5 Action Planning

Each person should be able to use the knowledge they have acquired so far to formulate an action plan for changing behavior(s). Action plans should contain specific goals and should identify sources of social support, possible barriers to making the change, and strategies for solving/overcoming each barrier. Goals and plans should be determined by the participant (the ball really has to be in their court at this point – if the patient does not "own" the plan, it is highly unlikely to be acted on. Of course, you can still give them prompts or advice if they want it).

Possible behavior change techniques
- Make a written action plan using the principles of SMARTER goal-setting (see Chap. 6).
- Focus on behaviors (what they will change) rather than outcomes (e.g. how much weight they will lose) for goal-setting.
- Set graded tasks (e.g. short-term and long-term goals). Small changes make a big difference over time, and the aim here is to move toward a *sustainable* change in energy balance (more energy out through physical activity and less energy in through changes to diet).
- Make the plan realistic – crash dieting does not work (weight goes back on because the changes made were not

sustainable) – you have to think about making changes for life – changes that you can live with! The aim should be to find a lifestyle that is both healthy and enjoyable (if it is not, then it will not be maintained).
- Prompt self-monitoring (of behavior and outcomes) as part of the plan.
- Include a coping plan (what will stop you and what can you do about it). This is sometimes called an IF-THEN plan (IF this happens, THEN I will do this).
- Include social support in the plan (who might be able to help you? What could they do?).

7.2.6   Self-monitoring and Reviewing Progress

There is clear evidence that people who monitor their weight or their physical activity are more successful at making and sustaining changes in diet and physical activity [1]. So patients should be strongly encouraged to monitor their progress in making changes on a regular basis. Of course, keeping food diaries is quite onerous, but this might be a useful thing to do once or twice to increase awareness of exactly what and how much is being eaten on a day to day basis. Patients can also keep track of their progress by using devices like pedometers, keeping track of their energy levels and mood, or just by mentally monitoring their ability to make the changes they have planned.

Progress against the goals set should be reviewed whenever possible at future meetings/consultations. It can also be useful to revisit the patient's motivation (which might change over time) and the usefulness or otherwise of their social support. A crucial aspect of the progress review is how to deal with setbacks, and this is dealt with separately below.

Possible behavior change techniques
- Prompt self-monitoring of behavior (and outcomes). This may involve the use of pedometers or self-weighing or occasional use of food or activity diaries.

- Provide feedback on performance. If there is success, celebrate it! – ask the patient how they feel about their progress and then add your own praise. If there have been problems, then use "relapse management" techniques to address them (as below).
- Review and reset goals (if a goal has been achieved, then consider adding new goals or increasing the level of change).

7.2.7   Managing Setbacks

The normal way that human beings learn anything is to learn from experience, and learning how to succeed with behavior change is no exception – *it is a process of trial and error*. You can help your patients to learn from their experiences with behavior change how to build on success and how to manage setbacks or new challenges. The idea is to help them to use the feedback from their ongoing experience of making behavioral changes to revise their action plans and strategies for change. It is important if people have not succeeded to stop this from resulting in a loss of confidence. To do this you need to "reframe" failure – explain that it is normal not to succeed at the first attempt – in fact most people take six or seven attempts before they succeed in losing weight or stopping smoking. The key to success is to see this as a process of trial and error and to learn from this setback – what went wrong and what could you do differently next time to stop this happening again? Each setback is not in fact a failure, but a valuable learning opportunity! If you can learn from the setback, you will be better equipped to reach your goal at the next attempt.

Possible behavior change techniques
- Reframe "failure" as a learning opportunity (as above). Explain that it is normal to have setbacks and/or to make several attempts in order to succeed.

- Problem-solving – help the patient to figure out what stops him/her from succeeding (or what circumstances are associated with relapses) and what can be done about this going forward.
- Review and reset goals: If the patient has already tried several strategies without success, maybe the goal is not right and a different dietary change or activity might be easier/more achievable at this stage.
- Provide information (Ask-Tell-Discuss).
- Review action plan (especially the coping plan).

7.3   Share the Work

You are not the only person who can support your patient and you are certainly not the biggest influence in their lives. So why not think about how you can pass on some the workload to other influential people in the patient's world? One possible resource is the patient herself/himself – can they do some of this for themselves? It can be useful to give the patient "homework" in-between sessions – this can consist of reading up on healthy eating/other important information, keeping food or activity diaries, making action plans (based on forms you can supply), and keeping track of what are the major challenges or barriers that crop up over a period of time (so you can discuss them next time you meet). A major advantage of getting the patient to share the workload is that it helps to get him/her to "own the problem."

You can also encourage the patient to engage social support from family and/or friends, as I have described above, this is a very powerful and important technique.

Other people either within the surgery (e.g. healthcare assistants) or within your local community (volunteers) may be able to help, especially if appropriate training can be provided.

7.4   Use Your Resources Wisely

In healthcare practice, time is always a scarce resource, and so it is useful to think about how this type of complex intervention can be delivered with less time or resources. You could consider:

(a) Spreading intervention over several sessions.
(b) Working with groups of patients. If you set up groups, instead of using one-to-one advice, then 6 h of group work, treating ten patients uses less time (360 moin) than seeing them each for 10 min on 6 occasions (600 min). Not only that, but each patient then gets 6 h of treatment time, instead of just one and this is more like the kind of time they need to properly plan and monitor and learn how to succeed in making lifestyle changes. Evidence shows that groups work just as well as individual interventions.
(c) Using the practice database to set reminders/repeat appointments. Reviewing progress over time (building on their experiences over time) is a key factor, and so having a systematic approach to follow up is important.
(d) Engaging the help of others (as above).

7.5   Keep Notes

Although it can seem to be a drain on time to make notes, in the ongoing encounter needed to support behavior change, this can actually save time. Keeping notes on basic ideas covered at each session will prevent you from having to recover old ground the next time you see the patient. You might consider using the practice database (or other source) to record:

(a) The patient's main motivation/reason for wanting to make a change
(b) What they went away planning to do – any goals they set
(c) Possible barriers to change

(d) Any ways to overcome barriers that they identified
(e) Any ideas for engaging other people to support them
      (who are they; what help could they provide)

7.6   Get Skilled Up

Good training is available for supporting behavior change. Ask yourself whether you are confident in each of the following key skills, and if not, think about seeking training to update your skills:

How confident are you that you can:

- Engage the patient: Using reflective listening and other patient-centered counseling techniques to engage the patient and build a sense of empathy (e.g. motivational interviewing skills such as reflective listening, affirmation, rolling with resistance). You need to be able to get the patient to be the person who decides whether to make changes and kind of activity/dietary changes are right for them.
- Exchange information: Using the Ask, Tell, Discuss technique.
- Explore and enhance the motivations of your patients: Exploring the pros and cons of making changes and their level of confidence about being able to succeed and use further techniques to build perceived importance and confidence.
- Use relapse prevention and problem-solving techniques to increase the chances of success.
- Put all these techniques together into a coherent plan/ sequence that you can adapt for each patient (as in the model above).
- Manage groups of people to ensure a positive group interaction.

7.7   Summary

Changing behavior is a journey – a difficult journey beset with pitfalls and obstacles. Having good intentions is not enough – you also need a plan. The only way to succeed is to first have a clear, strong reason (motivation), then to develop a clear, specific plan of action (including a plan of what you are going to do, who is going to help you (social support), and how you are going to overcome any likely obstacles), then to carefully monitor what works and what does not work so that you can learn from experience. It is very important to realize that this is a process of trial and error and that you should not always expect to succeed straight away – you need to see it as a learning experience and if you do not at first succeed, keep going! With the right tools and strategies and the right training and a reasonable amount of resources, you can offer your patients a professional service that will maximize their chances of success. The key is to put the patient in charge and to take it a step at a time – encourage experimentation, but aim for sustainable changes that people can live (a healthy lifestyle that the patient can also enjoy) – these are more likely to be changes for life.

7.8   Resources

The Diabetes Prevention Toolkit: http://www.image-project.eu/default.aspx?id=17

Motivational Interviewing Network of Trainers: http://motivationalinterviewing.org

Shaping Up: Weight loss intervention materials and training: http://www.shape-up.org/contacts.html

Diabetes self-management training:
http://www.xperthealth.org.uk/
http://www.desmond-project.org.uk/

Let's Get Moving: A Department of Health funded initiative/training on using brief interventions in a practice setting to help promote physical activity. The Let's Get Moving information pack can be downloaded from: http://www.bhfactive.org.uk/sites/Exercise-Referral-Toolkit/links.html

Diabetes Prevention Network: http://nebel.tumainiserver.de/dp/

References

1. Greaves CJ, Sheppard KE, Abraham C, Hardeman W, Schwarz P, Roden M, et al. Systematic review of reviews of intervention components associated with increased effectiveness in dietary and physical activity interventions. BMC Public Health. 2011;11:119.
2. Lindström J, Neumann A, Sheppard K, Gilis-Januszewska A, Greaves CJ, Handke U, et al. Take action to prevent diabetes: a toolkit for the prevention of type 2 diabetes in Europe. Horm Metab Res. 2010;42:S37–55.
3. Greaves CJ, Reddy P, Sheppard K. Supporting behaviour change for diabetes prevention. In: Schwarz P, Reddy P, Greaves CJ, Dunbar J, Schwarz J, editors. Diabetes prevention in practice. Dresden: TUMAINI Institute for Prevention Management; 2010. p. 19–29.
4. Rollnick S, Mason P, Butler C. Health behaviour change: a guide for practitioners. Edinburgh: Churchill Livingstone; 1999.
5. National Institute for Health and Clinical Excellence. Obesity guidance on the prevention, identification, assessment and management of overweight and obesity in adults and children. London: National Institute for Health and Clinical Excellence; 2006.

Index

Printed by Printforce, the Netherlands